Healing, Disease and Placebo in Graeco-Roman Asclepius Temples

Advances in the Cognitive Science of Religion

Series Editors
Armin W. Geertz Aarhus University
Jesper Sørensen Aarhus University
Valerie van Mulukom Coventry University

This series seeks to publish empirical, experimental and theoretical studies in the cognitive science of religion. Cognition is here broadly conceived as consisting of both internal and bottom-up processes on the one hand and external, extended, materialized and top-down processes on the other. This series is committed to a conception of human beings as highly social, embodied, embrained and enculturated organisms. Therefore, studies that emphasize any or several of these aspects are welcomed.

This series incorporates the series Religion, Cognition and Culture, formerly published by Routledge, and is associated with the *Journal for the Cognitive Science of Religion*, the official journal of the International Association for the Cognitive and Evolutionary Sciences of Religion.

Healing, Disease and Placebo in Graeco-Roman Asclepius Temples

A Neurocognitive Approach

Olympia Panagiotidou

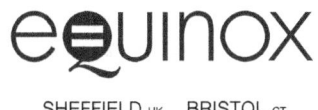

SHEFFIELD UK   BRISTOL CT

Published by Equinox Publishing Ltd.

UK: Office 415, The Workstation, 15 Paternoster Row, Sheffield, South Yorkshire S1 2BX

USA: ISD, 70 Enterprise Drive, Bristol, CT 06010

www.equinoxpub.com

First published 2022

© Olympia Panagiotidou 2022

All rights reserved. No part of this publication may be reproduced or transmitted in any form or by any means, electronic or mechanical, including photocopying, recording or any information storage or retrieval system, without prior permission in writing from the publishers.

ISBN-13 978 1 80050 141 6 (hardback)
        978 1 80050 142 3 (paperback)
        978 1 80050 143 0 (ePDF)
        978 1 80050 168 3 (ePub)

British Library Cataloguing-in-Publication Data

A catalogue record for this book is available from the British Library.

Library of Congress Cataloging-in-Publication Data
Names: Panagiotidou, Olympia, author.
Title: Healing, disease, and placebo in Graeco-Roman Asclepius temples : a neurocognitive approach / Olympia Panagiotidou.
Description: Sheffield, South Yorkshire ; Bristol, CT : Equinox Publishing Ltd, 2022. | Series: Advances in the cognitive science of religion | Includes bibliographical references and index. | Summary: "This book follows the evidence for Asclepius' supplicants from the moment in which they realized that they were sick until the healing experiences, which they might have had at the asclepieia. From a historical perspective, the main features of the Asclepius cult, as they were shaped mainly in the Hellenistic and Roman periods, are examined"—Provided by publisher.
Identifiers: LCCN 2021046030 (print) | LCCN 2021046031 (ebook) | ISBN 9781800501416 (hardback) | ISBN 9781800501423 (paperback) | ISBN 9781800501430 (pdf) | ISBN 9781800501683 (epub)
Subjects: LCSH: Asklepios (Greek deity)—Cult. | Healing--Religious aspects. | Medicine, Greek and Roman.
Classification: LCC BL820.A4 P36 2022 (print) | LCC BL820.A4 (ebook) | DDC 292.2/113—dc23/eng/20211123
LC record available at https://lccn.loc.gov/2021046030
LC ebook record available at https://lccn.loc.gov/2021046031

Typeset by JS Typesetting Ltd, Porthcawl, Mid Glamorgan

For Nikos and Melia ...

For Zafeiris and Maria ...

Contents

	Figures	ix
	Acknowledgements	xi
	Introduction	1
1	Setting the Theoretical Framework	21
2	Forming Ideas about Asclepius and His Healing Power	37
3	The Spread of the Asclepius Cult: Deciding to Visit an *Asclepieion*	67
4	Taking the Journey: Arriving at the *Asclepieia*	91
5	The Culmination of Incubation: Creating the Miracle	123
	Conclusion: Completing the Loop	153
	References	161
	Index	203

Figures

1. Statue of Asclepius from the *asclepieion* of Epidaurus — 46
2. The stoa of *abaton* at the *asclepieion* of Epidaurus — 78
3. The brain: reward system and social learning — 88
4. The *asclepieion* of Kos — 96
5. Mesolimbic dopamine system — 108
6. Votive relief with an inscription dedicated to Asclepius and Hygeia — 110
7. Votive terracotta to Asclepius, fourth century BCE — 120
8. Model of the *asclepieion* at Epidaurus, Greece, 1936 — 124
9. Votive relief of Asclepius healing a patient — 132
10. The dreaming brain — 138

Acknowledgements

Writing this book was a long journey, during which some important people contributed in one way or another to move forward, to overcome obstacles and to reach the final destination that is this publication.

From the conception of the original idea of this book to its final publication, Armin W. Geertz, professor at Aarhus University, was the motivator in every step of the way. I'm deeply grateful for his trust, guidance, patience and manifold help during my research and writing, and then for the decisive role he played for having this book published. His encouragement was crucial every time I confronted obstacles and felt disappointed.

A special gratitude I owe to Professor Anders Klostergaard Petersen from Aarhus University for reading the whole manuscript, even in hardship, and provided me with valuable feedback. His constructive criticism helped me approach in more depth some major theoretical issues and to theoretically enhance my arguments.

I would like to express the deepest appreciation to my teacher at the Aristotle University of Thessaloniki, Professor Panayotis Pachis, for the opportunities he offered me, since I decided to work on cognitive approaches to ancient cults, and Asclepius in particular. His ideas and constructive comments as well as his encouragement often helped me overcome myself. Without his extensive help, this adventure in the field of the Study of Religion would never have started.

I am deeply grateful to Professor Luther H. Martin from the University of Vermont for supporting me in sailing the unchartered waters of cognitive historiography. He provided me with the guidance, motivation and instruction to press on through the many frustrating times.

I would also like to thank Professor Roger Beck from the University of Toronto. His work and writings as well as our discussions were priceless in shaping my thought and my research.

I also wish to thank Dimitris Xygalatas (associate professor of anthropology at the University of Connecticut), Aleš Chalupa (assistant professor of the study of religions at Masaryk University), Yulia Ustinova (professor of general history at Ben-Gurion University of Negev) and Aggeliki Ziaka (assistant professor at the School of Theology of Aristotle University of Thessaloniki), who all read the original manuscript and provided me with comments and suggestions, which broadened my perspective and way of thinking.

Furthermore, I would like to acknowledge the financial and academic support of Aarhus University. I'm deeply indebted to the Faculty of Arts for granting me a scholarship in order to pursue my research in cognitive theories in Denmark and for giving me the opportunity to edit and polish the original manuscript some years later. Without this contribution the completion of my research and this publication would have been impossible. Special thanks I also owe to the members of the Religion, Cognition and Culture Research Unit (RCC) for their valuable ideas and suggestions during our meetings every Thursday during the fall semester of 2011–2012.

I would also like to acknowledge that the last part of my research and final amendments and editing of the manuscript was co-financed by Greece and the European Union (European Social Fund- ESF) through the Operational Programme 'Human Resources Development, Education and Lifelong Learning' in the context of the project 'Reinforcement of Postdoctoral Researchers – 2nd Cycle' (MIS-5033021), implemented by the State Scholarships Foundation (IKY).

Some preliminary ideas of my research were presented and shaped during a series of conferences and workshops which took place at the Aristotle University of Thessaloniki (the 3rd Annual Student Conference of the Study of Religion and Sociology and the conference Explaining Religion: Method, Theory & Experiment), at the Alexandria Center of Hellenistic Studies (2nd Hellenistic Studies Workshop), at the Masaryk University (Past, Present, and Future in the Scientific Study of Religions, Workshop by the Laboratory for the Experimental Research of Religion (LEVYNA), the Czech Association for the Study of Religions (CASR) and the Department for the Study of Religions, Masaryk University), in Ebeltoft, Denmark (Conversion and Initiation in Antiquity: Shifting Identities – Creating Change), in Loutraki, Greece (Spatializing Practices: Landscapes, Mindscapes, Socioscapes. Towards a Redescriptive Companion to Graeco-Roman Antiquity), at the University of London (Ancient Religions and Cognition Workshop by the University of Liverpool) and at the

Columbia University, USA (Popular Medicine in the Graeco-Roman World). I wish to thank the organizers of these conferences and workshops for their invitations. Special thanks are due to Panayotis Pachis, Thanasis Koutoupas, Lee McCorkle Jr, Dimitris Xygalatas, Luther H. Martin, Roger Beck, Nickolas Roubekas, Esther Eidinow, Tom Harrison and William V. Harris for the opportunities they gave me to present my research and to receive valuable feedback and ideas from the participants in these conferences and workshops.

I would also like to thank my friend and colleague, Spiros Piperakis, for our discussions and shared interests during our Master and PhD studies.

I owe special thanks to my family. Words cannot express how grateful I am to my father, Zafeiris, my mother, Maria, and my brother, Vasilis, for their love, all the sacrifices they've made on my behalf and their support during all the moments of disappointment and anxiety. I thank them because they never lost their optimism, even when I lost mine, they never stopped believing in me, even when I stopped believing in myself, and they are happier than me with my every little or big step.

Last but not least, I thank Nikos and Melia. I need to express my thanks to Nikos for being my best friend, my most severe reviewer, the most enthusiastic supporter of my work, my mate. He was beside me in all the difficulties, he supported me in the frustrations, he shared my concerns, he delighted with my ideas and never resented the long periods we needed to stay away. And I thank our daughter Melia for filling my every day with smiles and love. I hope that this book would be one more reason for her to feel proud of her mom.

For these and so many other reasons, this book is dedicated to my beloved persons. Sharing your joy with your beloved persons is the greatest happiness.

Introduction

A Cognitive Historiography of the Asclepius Cult

This book sets out to narrate a story of religious healing that took place at sanctuaries dedicated to the ancient Greek god Asclepius, the so-called *asclepieia*. The main characters in this narrative are the supplicants who were afflicted by various illnesses or diseases[1] and sought the help of Asclepius.

The Asclepius cult developed into a religious institution of Greek antiquity, which mainly ministered to people with health problems. It appeared in Greece in the sixth century BCE, thrived especially in the Hellenistic period, spread throughout the Graeco-Roman world and continued to flourish until the final dominance of Christianity in the fifth century CE. In the Classical period, the most significant *asclepieia* were constructed in Epidaurus in Peloponnese, Pergamum in Asia Minor, Lebena on Crete and on the island of Kos.[2] From the Hellenistic era onwards temples of Asclepius were built in most cities of the Graeco-Roman world.

People used to pray to Asclepius for the maintenance of their health and their families' well-being. When individuals were afflicted by illnesses or diseases, they could visit the local Asclepius sanctuaries to ask for recovery. However, when patients were able to travel and could afford the expenses, they could visit one of the great *asclepieia* where the god's healing abilities were considered to be more direct and effective. These sanctuaries gradually developed into important healing centres and attracted visitors from far and near. The supplicants arrived at the great *asclepieia* expecting direct communication with the god during the ritual of incubation

---

1. More extensive discussions of the terms and of the distinction between 'illness' and 'disease' follow in Chapter 1.
2. For the sake of brevity, these sanctuaries are called great *asclepieia* throughout this study.

(ἐγκοίμησις)[3] that constituted the main cult practice in which Asclepius appeared to perform treatments.

Many inscriptions unearthed in the *asclepieia* preserve personal stories of healing that supplicants of Asclepius claimed to have experienced during their visits to the sanctuaries. The collections of the so-called *iamata* (ἰάματα) from the Epidaurian *asclepieion* (*IG*² IV, 1, 121–122) as well as the healing inscriptions uncovered in the sanctuaries of Pergamum (*IPerg.* II) and Lebena (*I.Cr.* I) constitute the best-preserved testimonies of Asclepius' supplicants. In all likelihood, it would have been the priests at these sanctuaries who transcribed the stories into a written form that could be displayed (see, for example, LiDonnici 1992, 28–38, 1995, 65–69; Van Straten 1992, 253–254; Martzavou 2012, 177, 185). These inscriptions provide information about the health problems from which the supplicants suffered, the applied therapeutic methods and the latter's potential health outcomes. Many of the stories that can be pieced together from the inscriptions were probably originally circulated by word of mouth among people of the Graeco-Roman world, and it is likely that these stories contributed to the spread of Asclepius' reputation (cf. LiDonnici 1992, 29, 35).

Many of the healing inscriptions found at the *asclepieia* are still readable today, and form the main sources for modern research. German archaeologist Rudolf Herzog was the first to collect the Epidaurian healing inscriptions in his book *Die Wunderheilungen von Epidauros ein Beitrag zur Geschichte der Medizin und der Religion*, published in 1931.[4] Some years later, Lynn R. LiDonnicci collected the votive inscriptions of the Epidaurian *asclepieion* and quoted them in the original and in English translation in his monograph, *The Epidaurian Miracle Inscriptions* (1995). LiDonnicci studied the wider archaeological contexts in which *iamata* were found, investigated

---

3. Ludwig Deubner was the first who studied the ritual of incubation in his dissertation written in Latin in 1900; Mary Hamilton (1906) also studied the history of incubation from the ancient to modern era applying historical methods. Two recent studies also focus on the ritual of incubation. Hedvig Von Ehrenheim, in his work *Greek Incubation Rituals in Classical and Hellenistic Times* (2015), provides an illuminatig study on the ritual of incubation that framed the supplicants' requests or pursuits of a divinatory dream. Gil Renberg, in his two-volume work *Where Dreams May Come* (2017), offers a comprehensive study of the rituals of incubation in the ancient world based on the preserved literary sources; see also Patton 2004; Renberg 2006; Harrisson 2014.

4. Herzog quotes the *IG* no. 121–124, vol. IV, both in the original and in German translation. Based on the *iamata*, he studies the history of medicine and religious healing in the Graeco-Roman world.

the thematic and stylistic issues of the inscriptions, traced their source material and studied their chronological range, while he suggested possible processes and factors which would have affected the inscriptional production. However, the most monumental study of the Asclepius cult was offered in the mid-twentieth century by two philologists and researchers in the history of medicine, Emma and Ludwig Edelstein. The authors collected all the pertinent written testimonies and epigraphic records in the first volume of their work *Asclepius: A Collection and Interpretation of the Testimonies*, which they quoted both in the original and in English translation arranged by subject. Their work, published in 1945 and republished later, in 1998, represents the keystone study of Asclepius for many decades, and largely retains its value until today.[5] In 2005, the classical archaeologist, Jürgen Riethmüller, offered the almost exhaustive presentation of the archaeological evidence from the *asclepieia* along with a vast number of ancient sources and modern literature for each cult site in his two-volume study, *Asklepios: Heiligtümer und Kulte*. Although, his volumes could not replace those written by Emma and Ludwig Edelstein, they might be used as supplements, since they constitute the first integrated research in the archaeological remains from each known *asclepieion*.

The abundant written testimonies and archaeological evidence for Asclepius and his healing powers made the study of his cult a popular topic for historical research. Modern historians study the appearance of Asclepius in myths and narratives (e.g. Edelstein and Edelstein 1998, vol. 2; Kerényi 1959), the development of his healing cult into a religious institution (e.g. Riethmüller 2005, vol. 1) and the flourish of the cult in the local sanctuaries (e.g. Aleshire 1989; Melfi 2007), as well as its relationship to human doctors and Hippocratic medicine (e.g. Wickkiser 2008). In addition to the study of the Asclepius cult as an official religious institution, its essential relation to one of the most personal domains of human experience, that of health and disease, drew historians' attention to the individual experiences of patients who resorted to the *asclepieia* and contributed to the development and spread of the cult. In particular, historians have been interested in the reception of the healing inscriptions and anatomical votive offerings displayed in the sanctuaries by the supplicants as well

---

5. As the authors admit, they intentionally left out the archaeological evidence from their already voluminous work, since they believed that the material remains of the Asclepius cult would not offer further evidence to their study and conclusions.

as in the latter's feelings, emotions, and expectations during the ritual of incubation (e.g. Deubner 1900; Hamilton 1906; Meier 1967; Edelstein and Edelstein 1998, v. I, 142–180; Prêtre and Charlier 2009; Martzavou 2012; Błaśkiewicz 2014; Panagiotidou 2014a, 2021a, 2021b; Von Ehrenheim 2015; Renberg 2017; Molen 2019).

In addition to historians, the healing stories preserved on the inscriptions drew the attention of scholars from the fields of medical history and psychotherapy to the therapeutic methods and the psychological impacts and potential healings that supplicants could have experienced at the Asclepius sanctuaries during incubation. Mary Hamilton in her work *Incubation or The Cure of Disease in Pagan Temple and Christian Churches*, published in 1906, studied the similarities between incubation practised at the *asclepieia* and hypnosis applied in scientific medicine. Jungian therapist Carl Alfred Meier, in his book *Healing Dream and Ritual – Ancient Incubation and Modern Psychotherapy*, published in 1967, focused on the similarities between the curative methods employed by the ancient healing cults (i.e. the Asclepius cult) and the Jungian psycho-therapeutic methods, and explained mental illness and healing based on the common features of human nature. The French archaeologist Clarisse Prêtre and the doctor Philippe Charlier in their book *Maladies humaines, thérapies divines: analyse épigraphique et paléopathologique de textes de guérison grecs* (2009) investigated the medical information that can be found in 23 inscriptions from the *asclepieia* about the nature of the diseases from which the supplicants suffered, the therapeutic practices of Asclepius and their potential usefulness in comparison to the methods of the Greek and Roman doctors.

Furthermore, the massive number of healing narratives and the popularity of Asclepius during Graeco-Roman antiquity, testified by ancient sources and archaeological findings, raised the question in historical research about the possible effectiveness of the asclepian therapeutic treatments. Some scholars suggested that such treatments could have provided actual relief to suffering patients operating as a kind of placebo effect (e.g. Askitopoulou et al. 2002, 12; Lyttkens 2011; Martzavou 2012). Such suggestions assumed a biological phenomenon that has deep roots in human evolution and may provide a plausible explanation of the cult's flourish, but were not grounded on specific scientific evidence about the ways in which the Asclepius cult could have induced placebo responses to the patients.

The present study begins from the historical premise that the placebo effect could have played a role in healing at the Asclepius sanctuaries, and examines this plausibility in light of contemporary theories and neurocognitive research on placebo effects. The main aim is to explore the specific biological, cognitive, and psychological processes as well as the external cultural and social influences that would have shaped personal healing experiences and potential placebo responses of the supplicants. In particular, the evidence for Asclepius' supplicants is presented from the moment in which they realized that they were unwell to their return to health (or not) at the Asclepius temples. The historical evidence is supported by theoretical tools from the cognitive sciences that enable an examination of the preconditions, interactions and contextual conditions which might have generated placebo effects in Asclepius cult contexts. In that light, this study approaches Asclepius supplicants as biological, social, cultural and historical agents who had to cope with particular health problems, and who made use of available cultural heuristics, and it examines the likely impacts and influences of the Asclepius cult contexts on the bodies and minds of patients, which might have generated the 'healing miracles' at the *asclepieia* as a result of placebo effects.

From this perspective, this study applies a neurocognitive approach to the Asclepius cult that may shed light on the ways in which people of the Graeco-Roman world would have coped with the experience of sickness, and would have chosen to visit the *asclepieia*, where they might find relief of their health problems. Admittedly, many historians and classicists criticize cognitive approaches to ancient cults and past agents' minds. They argue that without direct contact with people, it is not possible to study their mentalities. Historians of religion instead focus their studies on the material remains and written testimonies left by the people of the era under investigation. Fieldwork, like that carried out by ethnographers and anthropologists, is not possible in the discipline of history (Panagiotidou 2014b, 16; Pachis and Panagiotidou 2017).

However, the narratives, written texts and material remains available for historical research may reveal much more than the stories they convey. Every text, artefact, painting, relief, coin, vase or architectural remain directly or indirectly refer to their creators, users and perceivers, implying multiple motives, purposes, knowledge, skills, designs and communication among their constructors, users and perceivers, and bear the meanings ascribed to them by these people (Panagiotidou 2014b, 16; cf. Rublack 2013, 43; Sutton and Keene, 2015). Thus, although historians are not able to enter into direct contact with the people who lived in the Graeco-Roman period, they approach the ideas, knowledge and perceptions of these people through their 'discourse' reflected in the written testimonies and the archaeological evidence.[6]

Historical research is interested in exploring the perceptions, purposes and motives of the composers, who recorded the events unfolding in their surroundings, reasoned about abstract notions and communicated their stories to readers as well as the cultural influences and conventions, economical constraints and practical restrictions in the production of texts and artefacts (Panagiotidou 2014b, 16). The cognitive sciences may provide to historians well-articulated theories and scientific evidence that support their conjectures, throwing light on the underlying cognitive processes that would have mediated people's perceptions, reasoning, decision-making and communication within specific cultural settings.

This study is a combination of a historical approach with the theoretical tools provided by neurocognitive research. In particular, the stories narrated by the inscriptions are not viewed as literal records of events that actually happened at the Asclepius sanctuaries. Historical research has indicated that the production of the healing inscriptions was affected by complex personal motives, institutional purposes, social interactions, decisions and actions taken by the supplicants, the priesthoods and the temple authorities, including patients' desires to express their gratitude and to offer dedications to Asclepius, the priests' intention to propagate Asclepius' healing powers through the written records of reputed personal healing experiences, occasionally hiring specialists to inscribe these stories, the availability of specific craftships, the formation of conventionalized types of inscriptions, the supplicants' economic capacities, and so on. This study is interested in exploring those neurocognitive processes that would have mediated patients' perception and conception of the inscriptions and of the wider cult context, and the likely impacts of the Asclepius cult components on the supplicants' ways of thinking, reasoning, emotional states, decision-making and actions that might have influenced their health conditions. In short, the likely perception and impact of the Asclepius cult on the patients' bodies and minds that could have activated placebo responses are what mainly matter in this study.

From this perspective, I examine how patients would have perceived, conceived and reasoned about the healing stories of miraculous cures, therapeutic practices (e.g. extreme surgeries) and Asclepius' appearances to his supplicants either in dreams or visions. Some of these stories tend

---

6. On 'discourse', see Lincoln 1989; Murphy 2000.

towards the extraordinary and supernatural, and people might likely have challenged the truthfulness of these claims. As we shall see, this seems plausible in light of Pascal Boyer's (2002) suggestion that humans share common basic intuitions about the world, and that these may be violated by counterintuitive concepts such as religious ideas about superhuman agents. From this perspective, the healing narratives included counterintuitive elements which would have contradicted people's intuitively accessible understanding of the world. However, taking into account Paul Veyne's notion of balkanization (1988), the belief in the superhuman power of Asclepius would have been dependent on the contexts in which people heard about the healing narratives. Patients' psychological conditions (e.g. despair, anxiety, fear of death) might have made some of them more amenable to believe in Asclepius and hope in recovery through divine intervention. In addition, individual dispositions towards supernatural agents (e.g. gods, heroes) might have affected patients' willingness to believe in the superhuman powers of Asclepius. Therefore, I suggest that the perception of the healing narratives might largely have depended on the psychological needs of people who were afflicted by illnesses and diseases, and being despaired by their health conditions, looked for reasons to believe in recovery. Thus, despite the conception of the inscriptions as specific *systems of strategic communication* which intended to propagate the healing power of Asclepius, I examine how the healing narratives might have impacted supplicants' affective, cognitive and mental states and, through these, promoted belief in Asclepius and the possibility of health improvement.

Of course, we cannot assume that all supplicants who visited the *asclepieia* would have experienced immediate relief or cure. It is possible that many of the patients left the sanctuaries without any change in their health condition. Even some of those who experienced immediate relief from the symptoms of their illnesses at the sanctuaries, could have relapsed after they returned home (Martzavou 2012, 195). In addition, I do not examine the cases of supplicants who visited the *asclepieia* asking for divine interventions on behalf of their sick relatives or friends (see, for example, Von Ehrenheim 2015, 96–97; Renberg 2017, 613–621). I mainly focus on the possible impacts that the major message, propagated by the cult about the healing power of Asclepius, would have had on the supplicants who would have been convinced about the potentiality of healing.

So, this book comprises a historical study of the Asclepius cult, embellished by theoretical insights into the human mind provided by neurocognitive sciences. In particular, it can be considered a *cognitive historiography*[7] of patients who visited the *asclepieia* as supplicants, which intends to show a pathway of cooperation between historians and cognitive scientists that may deepen our modern understanding of past minds and more generally of human cognition. I do not assert that my conclusions are definitive. What I hope to do is trace an idealized journey of the kind that might have been taken by the patients at the *asclepieia*, examine the potential impressions that supplicants might have had during their stay at the temples and their participation in the therapeutic practices that were claimed to offer a cure, and explore the possibility of patients experiencing actual health improvements as a result of placebo responses.

Approaching the Supplicants of Asclepius – A Cognitive Perspective[8]

The beliefs in Asclepius's healing powers, and the practices and rituals employed at the *asclepieia* were formed in the wider social, cultural, and religious contexts of the Graeco-Roman world. People who participated in the cult practices and expressed themselves through communication with each other, shared ideas, perceptions, memories, desires, hopes and expectations which in turn influenced and transformed the wider contexts of their lives. As already noted, the incubation ritual, supplicants' illnesses and diseases, the miraculous divine healings and medical treatments offered by Asclepius have seized the attention of those studying the affects of the Asclepius cult on a more personal level (e.g. Deubner 1900; Hamilton 1906; Meier 1967; Prêtre and Charlier 2009). However, these

---

7. *Cognitive Historiography* constitutes a new field in historical research which is currently under formation and has attracted historians interested in using cognitive theories and methods in order to approach ancient cults and religious behaviours. The *Journal of Cognitive Historiography* aims to prompt discussion among scholars from different disciplines on the application of cognitive approaches to ancient cults, and to promote collaboration between historians and cognitive scientists. The first issue of the *JCH* includes articles which apply cognitive approaches to ancient cults and religious phenomena; see further Beck 2014; Griffith 2014; Chalupa 2014; Lundhaug 2014; Pachis 2014; Panagiotidou 2014b; Slingerland 2014.

8. The basic ideas of this section were originally published in the first issue of the *Journal of Cognitive Historiography* (Panagiotidou 2014b).

studies have tended to be heavy on assumption but lacking in appropriate theoretical tools (Panagiotidou 2014b, 15).

Such theoretical tools that may provide glimpses into supplicants' personal experiences are provided in cognitive science research that studies various cultural and religious phenomena and practices and offers well-articulated theories of human behaviours. Cognitive science has emerged as one of the most promising scientific disciplines in the study of the human brain, cognition, culture and religion. Researchers in this area investigate the universal constraints in the formation of different cultural expressions, social constructions, political developments and religious behaviours that are imposed by the common factor underlying all of human history: human cognition, which is the product of the evolutionary history of the human species (Martin 2012, 47, 59).[9]

Human cognition first attracted the interest of scholars coming from the disciplines of linguistics and psychology in the 1950s.[10] Cognitive sciences advanced rapidly – an advance facilitated by developments in computer and information technology, memory research and brain imaging techniques – and by the end of the twentieth century developed into a broad interdisciplinary field. The multiple aspects of human cognition, including the physiology, structure and activity of brain, the phylogenetic and ontogenetic development of human cognitive capacities and their neurological constraints as well as their interrelation with the peripheral neural, chemical and hormonal bodily functions, became an important field in evolutionary biology, neuroscience, computer science, cybernetics and artificial intelligence as well as ethnography and anthropology (Martin 2012, 43, 46).

Besides the capacities, mechanisms and processes taking place within the brain itself, cognitive scientists recognized that human cognition is highly dependent on the interplay between brain structures and the external world (natural objects, artefacts, other persons, etc.). Both the external and internal bodily milieus send incessant stimuli to multiple

---

9. Luther H. Martin is the first scholar of Hellenistic (Graeco-Roman) religions who applied cognitive theories to the cults of that era. In this section, I mainly refer to his work which highlights the value of cognitive approaches to historical studies, and provides further references to cognitive theories and studies and the possible collaboration between scholars from the disciplines of history and the cognitive sciences.

10. For an introduction to the cognitive science of religion, see Geertz 2004, 347–400, 2016 and 2020. For a general introduction to cognitive approaches in the field of the study of religion, see Xygalatas 2006, 9–87 (in Greek); Martin 2012, 46–58.

brain regions, which process the sensory inputs and information in order to generate mental representations of the organism itself and various aspects of reality. A wide range of these representations are formed without reaching the level of consciousness, and allow humans to maintain their bodily physiological functions, orient themselves in space, interact with external objects and other persons, adopt particular intentions, and carry out their actions. Specific cognitive mechanisms, such as memory, learning and reasoning systems, generate further intentional representations which enable humans to perceive themselves in space and time, define their likes and dislikes, project their lives into the future and plan their actions towards specific goals. The unique human ability to represent own representations to others produces meta-representations which are transmitted among people, influence their own and others' perception and conception of the surroundings, excite the imagination, and constitute the ground for communication, sociality, culture and history.[11]

This wider conception of cognition promotes concilience and necessitates collaboration between neurobiology, the natural sciences and the study of human culture. Cognitive neuroscientists are currently interested in the impacts of cultural systems on brain structures, looking for 'cognitive universals' behind cultural, relativistic diversity (Roepstorff, Niewöhner and Beck 2010, 1051). In particular, cognitive scientists approach various religious traditions, practices and behaviours as aspects of human culture, and investigate the common cognitive capacities which lie behind seemingly different religious expressions.

Ethnographers and anthropologists, who study modern cultures and societies and approach religions as part of these structures, were the first to apply cognitive theories to religious phenomena and behaviours. The idea that religion could be approached in a scientific manner and viewed as a by-product of human evolution and culture was originally challenged by scholars of the disciplines of theology and the study of religion.

Despite the initial reactions and critiques, by the end of the twentieth century the application of cognitive theories to religious traditions, practices and beliefs has grown significantly, and subsequent years have seen an ever-increasing number of applied studies. Cognitive theories have also been articulated which focus on the universal aspects displayed in almost all religions – such as *religious rituals* (Lawson and McCauley 1990; McCauley

---

11. For a brief account of unconscious and intentional representations and meta-representations, see Martin 2012, 44–46.

and Lawson 2002), *religious ideas* (Guthrie 1992; Boyer 2002) and the *transmission of these ideas* (Sperber 1996; Whitehouse 2004) – and suggest their roots in common human biological functions (Martin 2012, 47–48).

Most recently, scholars have begun to look beyond biological explanations of the cognitive capacities behind the generation of religious beliefs, as these approaches were inadequate for understanding all the aspects and features of the various religious systems and traditions. Instead, scholars have looked for ways in which cognition is connected and interacts with the natural, cultural and social contexts of different regions and times.

Scholars at the Religion, Cognition and Culture Research Unit (RCC) in Aarhus University, in particular, investigate the interaction between the human brain, mind and body, and the external world. This research has led to valuable theories and approaches to multiple religious practices, rituals and behaviours (Geertz 2010, 304).

Armin W. Geertz (2010) has sketched out the terms of a biocultural theory which might induce a broader study of religion testable by cognitive scientists. His definition of religion as 'a cultural system and a social institution that governs and promotes ideal interpretations of existence and ideal praxis with reference to postulated transempirical powers or beings' (Geertz 1999, 471, 2010, 305) implies the essential interwoven aspects and units which compose and give meaning to various religious expressions. Religion is composed of beliefs, ideas and practices governed by specific principles and precepts similar to those of other cultural systems and social institutions. From this perspective, the findings of psychological and neurological studies of various cultural forms and expressions could similarly be applied to religion (Geertz 2010, 305).

According to Geertz, the first requisite for the creation as well as for the conception of culture, and therefore religion, is the brain. The brain, however, cannot exist without a body (Geertz 2010, 306). Through its *embodiment*, the brain forms an interactive system with the body that is composed of numerous complicated subsystems, each of which plays a crucial role in cognitive processes. Every alteration or stimulus from the internal or external milieu can impact the processes and functions taking place both in the brain and the body, and influence both bodily and mental states (Geertz 2010, 306–308).

Furthermore, although cognition develops and operates within the brain through its embodiment, it is not restricted to the body, but it is also *situated* via the body in the surrounding world (Geertz 2010, 308, 309; cf. Robbins and Aydede 2009, 30). It constantly perceives, manipulates and interacts with the surrounding environment, being 'extended' and 'distributed' to the external world (Geertz 2010, 309; cf. Hutchins 1995, 2010; Clark 1997, 2008; Rowlands 2003). Cognition is facilitated by the use of representations of the body and the external world in time and space (Geertz 2010, 310; Wilson 2010, 184). It further enables persons to voluntarily control their bodies and external objects which operate as 'cognitive anchors' for their minds enabling their cognitive development and re-organization (Geertz 2010, 309, citing Wilson 2010, 180–181; cf. Mithen 1996; Renfrew and Scarre 1998; Malafouris 2010). Humans phylogenetically evolved the ability to use their material environment, to create artefacts and to invent symbols which represent other objects or abstract notions.[12] These objects and representations – which are generated and are available in each culture – ontogenetically transform the ways in which cognitive processes unfold (Geertz 2010, 310, citing Wilson 2010, 180–181). Artefacts, symbols, metaphors, languages as well as buildings, art, literacy, music, rituals and other religious practices not only influence the '*contents* of cognition' (emphasis in the original), but also constitute essential 'cognitive components' which extend and distribute human intelligence beyond the borders of their biological brains and bodies (Geertz 2010, 310; cf. Norman 1993; Day 2004). In this view humans are *embrained* and *embodied* organisms *situated* in a specific world which provides various mind tools that 're-engineer cognition' (Geertz 2010, 310, citing Wilson 2010, 180–181).

Besides the interaction with their material and natural environment, humans interact with each other, and live in social groups. Their minds draw on collective networks of feelings, notions and ideas (Geertz 2010, 311), and evolve the ability to perceive the meaning of other people's bodily motions and gestures, facial expressions, gazes and tones of voice (Geertz 2010, 311; see Donald 2001, 256) – an ability that appears very early during ontogenesis, facilitates communication and further enables the development of culture (Geertz 2010, 311; see Donald 2001, 252–253). However, embodied and embrained humans not only generate specific cultural contexts. These contexts develop 'cognitive governance systems' which influence individual cognition and collective mentalities (Geertz 2010, 312), affecting the ways in which persons perceive themselves,

---

12. Various theories have been proposed regarding the stages of cognitive development (e.g. tool production, sociality, symbolic thought, language) during the evolution of the human species. See, for example, Donald 1991; Mithen 1996; for an overview of human cognitive evolution, see Hatfield and Pittman 2013.

others and the world. According to Merlin Donald (2001), 'cognitive governance systems' allow humans to tune themselves in with the available cultural models and to manage their bodies and minds following collective patterns of thought and behaviour being formed and promoted within specific cultural contexts (Geertz 2010, 311–313; cf. Donald 2001).

In particular, religion appears to be one of the most potent 'collective governance systems' (Geertz 2010, 312). Religions use higher order constructions of collective cognition such as myths, doctrines, rituals and other practices in order to manipulate people's minds and bodies and to influence their social identities and cultural worldviews (Geertz 2010, 313). They develop specific techniques that affect the lower order cognitive functions (emotions, learning, information processing, etc.), and embed their worldviews, patterns, categories and networks in people's minds. Religious norms, rules and patterns of behaviour 'are installed' in myths, rituals, systems of categorization, cosmologies and other constructions, and constitute 'higher order cognitive products' which impact the formation of identities and emotion regulation systems (Jensen 2010, 326–327). Especially during rituals, the religious precepts, norms and scripts of actions are invested with exceptional *emotional significance*[13] which promotes their internalization by individuals (Jensen 2010, 326–328). Religious narratives play a crucial role in this process, for they transform 'virtual worlds' into tangible 'social realities' (Geertz 2010, 313; cf. Donald 2001, 295). They embed ontological axioms and reflections about the existence of humans, superhuman powers and the world, including revelations and imagery which govern the meanings and local epistemologies of each social and cultural context (Jensen 2010, 327).

The term '*normative cognition*', suggested by Jeppe Sinding Jensen (2010, 323; cf. Jensen 2013, 2016), encapsulates the processes through which the 'collective ... directed ... externalized ... creative ... imaginary' cognition is formulated and governed by shared social norms, cultural models and religious cosmologies. Individuals participate in religious practices and interact with each other and external institutions. During social interaction and communication, collective rules of behaviour, social norms and cultural models govern, affect, and modulate human cognitive functions which tend to be normative (Jensen 2010, 323; cf. Donald 2001; Geertz 2010, 312–313). Further, people reflect on the social rules, norms, and schemata of behaviours, express themselves and contribute to further

---

13. This dimension is included in the definition of religion by Clifford Geertz (1990, 90).

externalization, development and 'up-loading' of the collective norms to a shared 'database' of norms, forms and guidelines made available to other persons (Jensen 2010, 326–327).

In this perspective, culture and cultural demonstrations are not conceived as abstract models, simply adopted by individuals. They comprise the dynamic products of the coordination between individual brains with each other and the external world, and of social interaction which promotes the internalization of collective representations, beliefs, practices and worldviews. According to Andreas Roepstorff and colleagues (2010), people constantly perceive their surroundings and interact with each other. During social interaction, their neural networks and the external contexts form dynamic 'systems-in-action' which mutually influence each other and generate multiple 'patterns of practice'. Patterns of practice develop over time into higher order models which enable humans to tune in with their brains and bodies, and share common perceptions, classifications and anticipations of their surroundings. In this way, *cultural systems* are conceived as sets of *patterns of practice* which *extend* individual cognition in the physical, social and symbolic world, and frame people's personal events in terms of others' past similar experiences (Roepstorff, Niewöhner and Beck 2010, 1056–1057).

Especially religions as cultural systems-in-action which engage particular systems of beliefs and normative orders in interplay with neural networks, establish specific patterns of practice which enhance coordination between individual brains, and promote the embedding of common perceptions of themselves, others and the world. Persons participating in particular religious practices might tune in with both their minds and bodies, co-constructing and sharing a common perceptual reality which grounds personal beliefs and justifies choices, goals and actions in their wider life. In an incessant process of reflective interaction, individuals shape the patterns of practice, which in turn influence their emotional states, categorizations, expectations, reasoning and perception of their surroundings (Roepstorff, Niewöhner and Beck 2010, 1056–1057).

Therefore, human cognition besides being *embrained, embodied, extended and distributed*, is deeply *encultured*, and depends on shared networks of emotions, feelings, information, knowledge and memories (Geertz 2010, 313).

Based on this acknowledgment, Geertz (2010, 314) argues that a biocultural theory of religion should take into account the social aspects, symbolic constructions and cultural models promoted by each religious tradition along with the psychological, bodily and cognitive processes that mediate attraction and participation of adherents to these traditions. All these aspects play a crucial role, and contribute to the development and diffusion of various religious traditions as well as their impact and establishment in human cognitive and social communities (Geertz 2010, 312–313).

Given these theoretical premises, ancient cults and religious practices can be understood as being generated by specific cognitive abilities developed during the evolution of the human species. In particular, they were formed and transformed through a continual interaction between the *neural networks* of the individuals participating in them, and the *patterns of practice* shaped by the interplay of those *embrained, embodied* and *encultured* individuals with the specific material conditions, conceptual frameworks and *normative orders* installed in their context.

In historical study, the exploration of contexts is of crucial importance in order for a past institution, practice or event to be conceived in its own terms. However, the recognition that these contexts are not just external settings in which people were put to live, but were co-constructed by themselves who in turn were influenced by their external surroundings opens a path for the application of cognitive theories to ancient cults. As Luther H. Martin (2012, 21) put it, 'the fundamental architecture of human cognition is the product of our evolutionary history. The capacities and constraints characteristic of this organic architecture can, consequently, allow historians to discriminate between and to organize their data in ways consonant with differences in human cognitive processes rather than conflating such data as the singular product of a common time and place'.

From this perspective, cognitive approaches to past religions mostly serve as supplementary research, providing the theoretical and experimental tools to approach cognition and mentalities of people in direct interplay with material, conceptual, symbolic, etc. surroundings. When studying human agents who lived in a past era, these approaches therefore help enrich historical knowledge, they fill possible gaps in its sources and offer new explanations and interpretations of complex historical conditions and events.

This book proposes a cognitive approach to the Asclepius cult as a supplement to existing historical studies. Without dismissing the findings of modern historical research, it aims to deepen understanding of the role of individual *reflective and normative cognition* in the spread of the religious precepts and beliefs in Asclepius, in the formation of the major structures of the cult and the establishment of specific *patterns of practice*. Furthermore, it uses the findings of modern research on placebo effects to investigate the mechanisms which motivated people to visit *asclepieia* and participate in the therapeutic rituals, and perhaps experience healing through placebo responses.

Cognition and History Meet at the Asclepius Temples – Outline of the Study

In this book, I examine how the context of the Asclepius cult, the various rituals and the medical treatments applied at the *asclepieia* could all have contributed to successful health outcomes for the patients. In this framework, I begin with the major premise that the Asclepius cult could have been a case of *placebo effects,* and I proceed to investigate whether the treatments and cures, which might actually have happened at the Asclepius sanctuaries, could have been the results of supplicants' placebo responses.

The notion of placebo effect is more thoroughly examined in Chapter 1. This chapter begins with a clarification of terms such as disease, illness and sickness, cure and healing as used in the study. In addition, a distinction is made between the use of the terms 'placebos' and 'placebo effects' in modern research. The physiological processes and mechanisms of placebo effects are then briefly outlined. The theory of placebo effects as articulated by Nicholas Humphrey (2002, 2005) is presented as the general theoretical framework for approaching healing at the Asclepius sanctuaries.

The Asclepius cult – following Armin Geertz's (2010, 304; cf. 1999, 471) definition of religion – developed into a particular 'cultural system and social institution' in the Hellenistic and Graeco-Roman era. Its main ideas, beliefs and precepts – which referred to the supernatural powers of Asclepius – as well as the healing practices applied at the *asclepieia* were formed and influenced by the wider historical, cultural and social contexts of that period. The reconstruction of these contexts is a prerequisite for any study which aims to investigate the likely cognitive, affective and bodily reactions of patients who visited the *asclepieia*, and might have been cured through placebo responses. Therefore, the second and third chapters (Chapters 2 and 3) outline the cultural, social, religious and intellectual contexts which underlied the popularity of Asclepius and prompted patients to turn to the *asclepieia*. The Hellenistic and Graeco-Roman culture – as any culture according to Donald (2001, xiv) – was not simply a 'set of shared habits, languages and customs', but could be seen as 'a gigantic cognitive web, defining and constraining the parameters of memory, knowledge, and thought in its members, both as individuals and as a group'. Therefore, these chapters do not discuss significant issues of the historical research on the Asclepius cult such as its development into an official institution, its geographical diffusion, and the historical formation of its major components. They mainly provide the wider settings in order to follow the mental and bodily itinerary of patients from illness or disease to healing. Since the historical and cultural background is determined, the focus is transferred to the protagonists – the persons who lived in the Graeco-Roman world, and made the decision to ask for Asclepius' aid. In order to understand the thoughts, beliefs, emotions and reactions of the protagonists, this book examines the likely biological, cognitive and affective processes which might have governed their actions, and generated placebo responses. In particular, social interaction and the various cognitive processes which mediate the ascription of specific values to places and motivate people to share common beliefs, are examined as the underlying personal and interpersonal processes which inspired hopes in recovery and attracted thousands of visitors to the Asclepius temples.

Chapter 4 follows the patients' mental and bodily journey to the great *asclepieia*, and their arrival and experiences within the sanctuaries. Quinton Deeley's (2004) insights on Clifford Geertz's (1990, 90) definition of religion are presented in order to highlight the sensory and semantic routes through which religious ideas could be transformed into beliefs during the rituals taking place at the *asclepieia*. The 'motivational salience hypothesis' of dopamine function articulated by Shitij Kapur (2003) and its application to religious rituals by Deeley (2004) is used to explain the possible assignment of salience to supplicants' internal thoughts and to the external events happening in the wider cult context. In particular, some healing inscriptions narrate stories about otherwise neutral events which were perceived as Asclepius' interventions by his supplicants. Even if these stories were invented, similar attribution of salience to random events was promoted by the cult and could be possible in the wider cult context. The neurobiology of these salience attributions to otherwise neutral events is discussed in relation to Kent C. Berridge and Terry Robinson's (1998) hypothesis about dopamine release in the human brain. Beyond the rituals, the inscriptions and anatomical votive offerings as a means of priming and indirect suggestion are further examined in order to highlight the roles of these material constructions in the inducement of placebo responses.

Chapter 5 focuses on the ritual of incubation and the healing experiences that patients expected to have in the *abaton*. In particular, the mechanisms, which can transform peoples' hopes and expectations into actual healing dreams and visions that activate placebo responses, are examined. According to the theoretical model suggested by Howard Leventhal and his colleagues (1982), cognitive and emotional care practised by doctors can amplify the effectiveness of the employed medical methods. Ted Kaptchuk (2002) describes five factors that influence the positive outcomes of both active and inert medical interventions and contribute to the *placebo drama*. Following his theory, I suggest that Asclepius, the patients, the relationship between the divine physician and his supplicants, the nature of the latter's impairments, the employed or prescribed treatments and the ritual settings in which these treatments were performed are the major components of Asclepian therapy. Particularly, the performance of healings during supplicants' sleep brings to the fore the matter of dreaming and the use of dreams as diagnostic tools by the Hippocratic doctors. The Hippocratic theory of dreams is examined in light of modern evidence which attempts to throw light on this complex mental state. Modern studies on the dreaming brain have not reached definite conclusions. However, the evidence that does exist can highlight some aspects of the dreams that Asclepius' supplicants might have had at his sanctuaries. In particular David Kahn, Stanley Krippner and Allan Combs's (2000) research on the psycho-physiological and cognitive structure of dreams, Allan Hobson (1994), Allen Braun and his colleagues' (1998) considerations on the biological processes of dreaming, Allan Hobson and Robert Stickgold's (1994) study of dreaming in REM and nREM sleep, and PierCarla Cicogna and Marino Bosinelly's (2001) theoretical assumptions about consciousness during dreaming are briefly presented in order to suggest that the supplicants could have had the desired and expected healing dreams in the context of incubation. The inducement of an altered state of consciousness resembling dreams or visions during incubation is further examined as a potential result of direct or indirect suggestions received by patients during their stay in the sanctuary. Milton Erickson's model of therapeutic suggestion (Erickson, Rossi and Rossi 1976) is presented as a possible explanation of the abnormal experiences that supplicants might have had in the *abaton*. Ernest and Kathryn Rossi's (2007) neuroscience perspective underlines those biological, neural and behavioural factors which can generate mind-body healing miracles as a result of placebo effects. Furthermore, Lawrence Barsalou and colleagues' (2005) theory about the embodiment of mundane knowledge and simulation processes which might generate religious visions is used as a plausible explanation of the healing dreams and visions that Asclepius' supplicants might have had during incubation. The chapter concludes with daybreak and the incubants' exit from the *abaton*. In particular, the processes through which the healing experiences could be perceived as actual events are examined.

In conclusion, the main steps of the kind of journeys supplicants might have followed in order to experience the *asclepieia*'s placebo effects are briefly reviewed. Although this study does not intend to prove that patients were actually healed at the Asclepius temples, the structure of the cult and propagation of the healing power of the divine physician might indicate that the cult officials and priests did intuitively use the power of placebo effects (cf. Burnett 2015). The Asclepius cult was the product of the Graeco-Roman world, but its flourish and expansion were largely dependent on the common cognitive and emotional processes developed during human evolution. Thus, this case study of Asclepius intends to highlight how the application of cognitive theories to an ancient cult can deepen modern historical knowledge of the persons who participated in this cult.

Chapter 1

Setting the Theoretical Framework

The wide diffusion of the Asclepius cult throughout Greek antiquity and the attraction of numerous supplicants who sought healing at his temples have raised the historical question about the possibility of successful cures experienced by patients. Considering the abundant testimony about the treatments employed at the *asclepieia* and personal healing stories, we can surmise that at least some of the supplicants could have experienced actual cures and relief from their illnesses and diseases. Such an assumption cannot be explained scientifically by recourse to a concept of divine healing. It can be, however, examined if we take into account the findings and theories of modern research on placebo effects. Theories on placebo effects may provide scientific evidence and theoretical tools for supporting historical assumptions about the possible effectiveness of Asclepian medicine.

In this chapter, I briefly sketch out the major concepts of placebo effect theories and provide some definitions and clarifications of placebo terminology. In particular, I clarify the slight differences in the meanings of the words 'disease', 'illness' and 'sickness' as well as between the terms 'cure' and 'healing'. I further spell out the distinction between 'placebos' and 'placebo effect' that is extensively used in neurocognitive research. I briefly refer to the health problems that placebo effects can contribute to healing. Then I outline the model of placebo effect suggested by Nicholas Humphrey which I shall use as the wider theoretical framework for my study. Although the following ruminations may seem very technical in nature, it is crucial to explicate them, before I proceed to employ them for casting light on the extant sources of the Asclepius cult.

Placebo Effect: Terms, Definitions and Theories

In order to examine the healing properties of placebo effects, it is first helpful to draw a distinction between disease and illness (Kaptchuk, Miller and Colloca 2009, 523; cf. Panagiotidou 2021a, 2021b).[1] Disease is defined as a biological malfunction which disrupts the physiology of the human organism (see Twaddle 1994, 8-9; Hofmann 2002, 652; Kaptchuk, Miller and Colloca 2009, 523; cf. Sisti and Caplan 2017). The symptoms which may be generated by the pathophysiology of a disease, like pain, hardship or exhaustion, are experienced as illness by the person (see Twaddle 1994, 10; Hofmann 2002, 652-653; Kaptchuk, Miller and Colloca 2009, 523). In this light, illness is defined as the experience of the symptoms of a disease. Both disease and illness are localized in the body, but the perception of these states is distinctive (Kaptchuk, Miller and Colloca 2009, 523). On the one hand people can be afflicted by a disease but they experience no symptoms, while on the other hand some patients may suffer from an illness but there is no diagnosable bodily malfunction. Illness, however, is not a solely mental or subjective state. It is the way in which the state of the organism is experienced by the suffering person (Kaptchuk, Miller and Colloca 2009, 526). In most cases there is a dynamic interrelation between disease and illness which affects the organism and the person respectively (Kaptchuk, Miller and Colloca 2009, 523; cf. Cassell 1991, 49; Panagiotidou 2021a, 2021b).[2]

Illness is usually recognizable by others and may have certain social implications which determine the quality of sickness. A patient is considered to be sick as long as he or she experiences the symptoms of an illness. Sickness is signified by accompanying social dysfunctions. The person who is sick cannot accomplish his or her social and professional activities, and is often spatially restricted to his or her home, hospital or sanatorium (see Twaddle 1994, 11; Hofmann 2002, 653; cf. Panagiotidou 2021a, 2021b).[3] In addition, the cultural conventions and conceptions of certain illnesses

---

1. On the distinction between disease and illness, see further Parsons 1951, 1958, 1964; Twaddle 1968, 1994, 22; Eisenberg 1977; Kleinman 1988; Sachs 1988; Hofmann 2002, 2017; Sisti and Caplan 2017. On the concept of disease and other epistemological issues that pertain to philosophy of medicine see Solomon, Simon and Kincaid 2017.
2. As the physician Eric J. Cassell (1976, 48) has aptly pointed out: 'Disease, then, is something an organ has; illness is something a man has'.
3. The definitions of sickness, illness and disease have been adopted by the World Health Organization.

and diseases may influence the ways in which patients experience sickness and socially perceive, conceive and present their health condition as well as their social status and the ways others perceive them.[4]

Therefore, we can hold that disease comprises a biological phenomenon, illness pertains to the phenomenology of the disease[5] and sickness consists in the social and behavioural implications of illness (Hofmann 2002, 657). Because all three terms refer to negative conditions, the ways in which these conditions are perceived and experienced by patients may generate unpleasant feelings and sensations.

Eric J. Cassell (1982) has suggested a distinction between physical distress and suffering pertaining to the experience of diseases, illnesses and sickness by individuals. Physical distress may derive from all the negative and unpleasant symptoms of a biological dysfunction which may affect the patients' quality of life restricting their bodily capacities and functions. The patients may be in distress because of a dysphoric illness, but they can also suffer from a disease without symptoms. The negative feelings of anxiety, fear, hopelessness, despair and disappointment which may be generated and frame an illness or a disease and the negative prospects in personal integrity and social life entailed by sickness may increase the dysphoric experiences and may cause suffering in patients.[6]

In conformity with the conceptions and semantic connotations of the aforementioned terms, further distinctions can be made concerning the processes and actions taken for the restoration of health. Thereby, curing involves all those means, substances, methods, practices and treatments that are employed in order to resolve the biological malfunction, to eliminate a disease, to relieve the physical distress caused by an illness and to restore the appropriate condition of the inflicted bodily parts or organs. Healing, on the other hand, refers to the more personal experience of alleviating and transcending suffering by restoring the health of the patient's organism as a whole (Egnew 2005).[7]

---

4. For example, the stigmatization of mental illness may induce fear of social exclusion in patients (see Susser 1973; Illich 1976).
5. On the phenomenology of illness, see further Svenaeus 2014.
6. Similarly, to the distinction Cassell made between disease and illness (1976, 48), he observes that 'suffering is experienced by persons, not merely by bodies, and has its source in challenges that threaten the intactness of the person as a complex social and psychological entity' (Cassell 1982, 639).
7. Thomas R. Egnew (2005) presented an 'operational definition' of healing as 'the personal experience of the transcendence of suffering'. The scientific exploration of healing and

The experience of illness and recovery may further involve different modes of healing. Therefore, the dysphoric experience of an injury, a wound or affliction by an illness or a disease may be naturally relieved and the dysfunction gradually be cured through the autonomous bodily processes of health restoration. This kind of 'natural healing' involves all those physical and biological processes inherent in the human body which strive to constrain external afflictions and internal dysfunctions restoring the organism's appropriate internal condition. The medical interventions, remedies and prescriptions which are administered to patients to cure the biological malfunctions and disturbances of the bodily functions comprise the so-called 'technological healing' which may further activate and amplify the self-healing mechanisms of the human body. In addition, the effectiveness of both 'natural' and 'technological healing' may be eliminated or enhanced by the external stimuli and prospects of healing given during the clinical encounter between health-providers and patients. The role of this kind of 'interpersonal healing' can be crucial for the accomplishment of the desired health outcome (Kaptchuk, Miller and Colloca 2009, 528). Although the aforementioned modes of healing may independently mediate and be conducive to health restoration, the overlap between the two and particularly the involvement of the so-called placebo effect in the healing processes seems to amplify the effectiveness of the employed healing methods (cf. Panagiotidou 2021b).

The placebo[8] effect comprises an excessive form of cueing or priming. It refers to the spontaneous reaction of the human body which can be activated even by the mere view of doctors or medical interventions and urge the organism to strive against external invasions or afflictions by illnesses and diseases (Eisenberg 1977; Blum 1985, 420; Kaptchuk 2002; Kaptchuk, Miller and Colloca 2009, 518; Kaptchuk et al. 2010; Benedetti, Carlino and Pollo 2011; Benedetti and Amanzio 2011). The placebo effect is

---

its role in healthcare systems comprise the main research area of the Samueli Institute (www.siib.org), which determines healing 'as the process of recovery, repair and return to wholeness. It is the foundation for a vision of medicine where the focus is the alleviation of suffering, the enhancement of well-being and the treatment of chronic illness' (Jonas and Chez 2006, 517; cf. Jonas and Chez 2004, S-1).

8. The term etymologically derives from the Latin phrase 'I shall please', which was used by professional mourners who were hired to mourn at funerals in the fourteenth century. In *Quincy's Lexicum-Medicum* (1811), the term is used as 'an epithet given to any medicine adapted more to please than to benefit the patient' (de Craen et al. 1999a, 511). On the history of the term 'placebo', see further Shapiro 1964.

a psychobiological phenomenon which has direct or indirect pharmacological and/or psychological results that may be generated by both actual and inert medical interventions (Benedetti et al. 2005; Kaptchuk et al. 2010). Via the operation of the placebo effect, people who feel ill can start to recover immediately after they receive medical treatments or remedies well before these therapies have time to impact on their organisms, if indeed the medicines are effective at all (Eisenberg 1977; Blum 1985, 420; Humphrey 2005, 1). The placebo effect can relieve illnesses, but may also influence the pathophysiology of a disease, and control its development (Kaptchuk, Miller and Colloca 2009, 523–525).

One should draw a distinction between the placebo effect and the term placebos which is mostly used to define inert remedies (sugar pills, saline injection, etc.) (cf. Panagiotidou 2021b). Even mere words, gestures, symbols and meanings may operate as placebos affecting people's minds and cognitive processes (Gelbman 1967; Chaput de Saintonge and Herxheimer 1994; Crow et al. 1999, 2; Oken 2008, 2812; Benedetti, Carlino and Pollo 2011). Although placebos are bio-medically inert, they can have physical results through the placebo effect which depends on the person, his or her health-conditions and the particular circumstances under which the inert remedies are administered (Crow et al. 1999, 1; cf. Wilkins 1985). The power of placebo effects, however, is not restricted to placebos but can also mediate and amplify the effectiveness of actual medical interventions with definite healing properties (Kaptchuk, Miller and Colloca 2009, 519).[9] Therefore, placebo effects may enhance or even accelerate positive health outcomes in various contexts, from official medicine to alternative healing practices (Kaptchuk, Miller and Colloca 2009, 527–528).

In particular, 'interpersonal healing' seems to comprise a crucial condition under which placebo responses can be activated and largely

---

9. On the distinction between *placebo* and *placebo effect*, see Brody 1982; Moerman 1983; Wilkins 1985; Miller and Kaptchuk 2008. In order to avoid confusion, some scholars have proposed the term 'meaning response' instead of the 'placebo effect' (see Brody and Brody 2000; Moerman 2002). Kaptchuk, Miller and Colloca (2009), however, propose the term 'interpersonal healing'. Other terms have been proposed to describe this effect, including 'expectancy effect' (Crow et al. 1999) and 'context effects' (Di Blasi et al. 2001). However, since the terms 'placebo effect' and 'placebo response' prevail in biomedical terminology, these terms are also used here. On the use and interpretation of the term 'placebo' and 'placebo effect', see Shapiro 1969; Borkovec 1985; Grünbaum 1981; Brody 1985; Gotzsche 1994; Kienle and Kiene 1996; Crow et al. 1999, 1–2; Miller and Kaptchuk 2008; Kaptchuk, Miller and Colloca 2009, 519.

intensified by the healing encounter between doctor and patient. The way in which a treatment is applied or a certain drug is administered by physicians is defined as 'the ritual of treatment', and can affect the healing process (Kaptchuk, Miller and Colloca 2009, 519). Modern clinical experiments show that supportive verbal and non-verbal communication between healer and patient can generate immediate therapeutic outcomes (Rescorla 1988; Voudouris, Peck and Coleman 1990; Ader 1997; Montgomery and Kirsch 1997; Benedetti et al. 2006, 345–346; Klinger et al. 2007; Kaptchuk, Miller and Colloca 2009, 522; Porro 2009, 2–3) deriving even from the simulation of a treatment (Kaptchuk 2002; Kaptchuk, Miller and Colloca 2009, 522; Kaptchuk et al. 2010; Benedetti and Amanzio 2011).[10] Conversely, the presentation of potential side effects of the applied treatments and of finally undesired outcomes may have negative psychological or even physiological results which entail a patient's clinical worsening, and are defined as nocebo effects[11] (Colloca et al. 2008a, 211, 216–217; see further Crow et al. 1999, 1, 4, 35; de Craen et al. 1999a, 514; Flaten, Simonsen and Olsen 1999; Benedetti et al. 2006, 2007, 2011; Scott et al. 2008; Colloca et al. 2008a).

Placebos in Medical Practices: How the Placebo Effects Relieve Pain and other Illnesses and Diseases

From a historical and cultural perspective, traditional and alternative medicine, on the one hand, is hardly based on a scientific knowledge and understanding of diseases, and employs only a few treatments with actual therapeutic properties. Meanwhile, the effectiveness of these traditional healing methods probably derives from patients' placebo responses (Kaptchuk, Miller and Colloca 2009, 523; see further Benson and Epstein 1975; Kaptchuk 2002; cf. Panagiotidou 2021b). Modern medicine, on the other hand, scarcely takes into account the significance and usefulness of placebo effects in the administration of active drugs and surgeries. However, even as recently as the nineteenth century, doctors depended on placebo responses when advising treatments (see, for example, de Craen et al. 1999a). Their medical practices, involving among others purgation,

---

10. On the significance of verbal communication, see Sternbach 1964.
11. Nocebo effects can be traced for instance in numerous examples of the magical papyri that engage in conjurations against rivals and enemies.

puncture, cupping, bloodletting, heating, freezing and causing of shock, were mostly pharmacologically inert, if not harmful (Turk, Meichenbaum and Genest 1987, 75; Jopling 2008, xii–xiii; Turk and Genest 2013, 287–288; see Shapiro 1963). The successful outcomes of these practices largely depended on the patients' beliefs in doctors' authority, and placebo responses to the applied treatments. From this perspective, according to Arthur Shapiro and Elaine Shapiro (1997a, 2), the history of both alternative and scientific medicine is largely involved with the history of placebo effects (see also Czerniak and Davidson 2012).

Modern scientific research that compares responses to real and deceptive drugs, has confirmed the effectiveness of placebo effects,[12] especially in the treatment of pain. Pain is considered to be a particularly subjective sensory perception. Research in both clinical and experimental settings implies that placebo effects can bring significant pain relief.[13] In particular, the analgesic power of placebo effects seems to be based on the inhibition of pain transmission by the system of pain modulation localized in the cerebral cortex. Specific cortical regions, such as the anterior cingulate cortex and the dorsolateral prefrontal cortex, seem to be activated by placebos (Benedetti et al. 2011, 344; see further Petrovic et al. 2002; Wager et al. 2004). Then, according to Falk Eippert and his colleagues (2009a), the whole system of pain modulation is involved, including the hypothalamus, the periaqueductal gray and the rostroventromedial medulla (Benedetti et al. 2011, 344). This activation extends into the spinal cord where dorsal horn neurons can be further inhibited (Benedetti et al. 2011, 344; see further Eippert et al. 2009b). This pain modulating system is opioidergic, and may induce placebo analgesia through the activation of μ-opioid receptors (Benedetti et al. 2011, 344; see further Wager et al. 2004, 2006; Zubieta et al. 2005). The dopaminergic reward system, originating in the ventral tegmental area with projections of the dopaminergic neurons to the nucleus accumbens, seems also to be involved in the process of placebo analgesia (Benedetti et al. 2011, 344; see further Scott et al. 2007, 2008).[14]

---

12. Although modern scientific medicine viewed with suspicion and often rejected the placebo effects, today these effects are considered to be biological phenomena amenable to scientific research.

13. On the placebo effects on pain and distress, see, for example, Price et al. 1999; Benedetti 2009.

14. Placebo and nocebo effects are connected with reverse responses of the dopamine and endogenous opioids in brain networks related to reward systems (Benedetti et al. 2011,

Beyond pain relief, placebo effects can be effective in a broad range of diseases – for example, stomach ulcer (de Craen et al. 1999b; Moerman 2000), asthma (Kemeny et al. 2007; Kaptchuk et al. 2008), headache (Diener et al. 2008), epilepsy (Niklson et al. 2006), heart disease (Archer and Leier 1992), Parkinson's disease (de la Fuente-Fernández and Stoessl 2002a; Goetz et al. 2008), depression (Leuchter et al. 2002), anxiety disorders (Pierce et al. 1996; Schweizer and Rickels 1997), etc. – as well as in significant numbers of patients, when they receive active or inactive agents (Agras, Horne and Taylor 1982; Rabkin et al. 1990; Archer and Leier 1992; Crowe McCann et al. 1992; Buckman and Sabbagh 1993, 246; Amigo et al. 1993; de Craen et al. 1999b; Moerman 2000, 51–72; Asmar, Safar and Queneau 2001; Mayberg et al. 2002; Humphrey 2002, 257, 2005, 1; Benedetti et al. 2005; Zhang et al. 2008). The placebo effects reinforce 'natural healing', that is, immune responses to infections and antibody production as well as the cure of many other illnesses and diseases (Benedetti et al. 2011, 346; see Pacheco-Lopez et al. 2005, 2006). According to Andrew Weil (1995, 53 cited in Humphrey 2002, 257), 'people can get better from all sorts of conditions of disease, even very severe ones of long duration'.

The Cognitive and Biological Underpinnings of the Placebo Effects

People suffering from the unpleasant symptoms of illnesses and diseases visit doctors – or other kinds of healers and practitioners – and expect to receive some kind of treatment.[15] The belief that receiving a specific remedy or drug, or even going through a surgical intervention is going to generate recovery is induced through various means mentioned by Humphrey (2005, 2): conditioning (Kapthchuk 2002, 818; see, for example, Rescorla 1988; Voudouris, Peck and Coleman 1990; Ader 1997; Montgomery and Kirsch 1997; Benedetti et al. 2006, 345–346; Klinger et al. 2007; Porro 2009, 2–3; Vits et al. 2011; Vits and Schedlowski 2014), associative learning (e.g. Vits and Schedlowski 2014), verbal instructions (e.g. Sternbach 1964; Uhlenhuth 1966; Amigo et al. 1993; Flaten, Simonsen and Olsen 1999;

---

344); see Schweinhardt et al. 2009. On nocebo hyperalgesia as opposed to placebo analgesia, see, for example, Benedetti et al. 1997, 2006; Colloca and Benedetti 2007.

15. For the unpleasant experiences of illnesses and somatic injuries in Graeco-Roman antiquity, see, for example, Grmek 1989; Nutton 2005; Androutsos et al. 2008.

Kaptchuk 2002, 817–825; Kaptchuk et al. 2010; Benedetti and Amanzio 2011), rational arguments, magical reflections, trust in authority[16] and implicit social suggestions.[17] In parallel with these means, personal mental and emotional states as well as subjective attitudes play a crucial role in health outcomes (Humphrey 2005, 2).

Modern neuro-immunological research has revealed close connections between the central nervous system (CNS) and the immune system in the human body and this gave rise to the discipline of psychoneuroimmunology (PNI) – also called psychoendoneuroimmunology (PENI) – which explores the brain-immunity effects and their correlations with certain psychological processes (see, for example, Ader and Cohen 1985; Ader, Cohen and Felten 1995; Dunn 2005; Irwin and Vedhara 2005; Ousman and Kubes 2012). The release of several neurotransmitters triggered by internal bodily or external contextual stimuli appears to comprise crucial signalling pathways for both immune activation and deactivation, and the generation of placebo responses (Humphrey 2005, 2; Oken 2008, 2813). In particular, as we have seen in the case of placebo analgesia, endogenous opiates comprise a 'chemical pathway' which seems to mediate placebo responses that modulate the perception and sensation of pain (Humphrey 2005, 2–3). In addition to their role in pain relief, endogenous opioid systems seem to contribute to 'the regulation of inflammation, nausea, wound healing and antibody production' (Humphrey 2005, 2).[18]

In addition to the release of opioids in the human brain and body, placebo effects may involve various brain and neural networks, and signalling pathways activated by complex 'effectors', depending on the context in which they are generated, and the mode of learning anticipation deriving from this context (Oken 2008, 2814). In all cases, the central nervous system constitutes the major 'mediator' in the physiology of placebo effects, since it comprises the locus of learning mechanisms

---

16. On the human tendency to imitate and admire prestigious individuals, see, for example, Henrich 2015, 124–131.
17. For a review of the major theoretical approaches to placebo effects, see Colloca et al. 2008; Colloca and Miller 2011.
18. Placebo analgesia is involved in pain management, and at least some aspects of this effect depend upon endogenous opioid systems. Administration of naloxone blocks the release of opioids in the brain, and suppresses the placebo effects. About placebo analgesia, see, for example, Price et al. 1999; Petrovic et al. 2002; Colloca et al 2006; Zubieta et al. 2006; Wiech et al. 2008; Lui et al 2010. See, however, Else-Marie Jegindø and colleagues' neurocognitive studies on pain, prayer and the opioid systems (Fardo et al. 2015).

and mnemonic systems and coordinates the operation of sensorimotor, autonomic, immune and endocrine systems (Oken 2008, 2813). In addition to the physiology and neuro-immunological systems which mediate the placebo effects, humans have particular personal features that make them more or less receptive to specific stimuli which can activate the relevant biological and neural systems of placebo responses (Oken 2008, 2813; see further Crowe McCann et al. 1992; Shapiro and Shapiro 1997a; Kaptchuk 2002; Zubieta et al. 2006).[19] According to Oken (2008, 2813), 'the interaction between the learned associations of the clinical situation and the person's particular biology' can induce a placebo effect, which is equivalent 'to a basic physiological process, such as modulation of sensory processing, release of neurotransmitters or alterations in hypothalamic–ituitary–adrenal axis or immune system activity'. The placebo response, in this way, is a multiple physiological procedure combining internal chemical and biological conditions, cognitive and perceptual processing and mood alterations (Oken 2008, 2813).[20]

In particular, associative learning and behavioural conditioning seem to comprise crucial cognitive processes which mediate the activation of placebo responses. In Pavlovian conditioning, neutral and inactive stimuli, such as inert drugs, assimilate or mimic active medical interventions which the patients have previously gone through. Thereby, previous experiences and learned information about unconditioned stimuli – that is, physiologically relevant stimuli (Hucklebridge 2002, 326) – are associated with and transferred to conditioned placebos – that is, physiologically neutral stimuli – activating similar immune responses with those generated by active remedies and treatments (Oken 2008, 2813; Benedetti et al. 2011, 346; see further Siegel 2002). Experimental research seems to confirm that behavioural conditioning plays a significant role in the activation or inhibition of the immune system and the generation of

---

19. According to Lasagna et al. (1954), anxious individuals are more amenable to placebo responses. Anxiety seems to be connected with placebo responses, according to Tibbets and Hawking 1956 and Medvedev et al. 1984. McNair et al. 1979 and Pichot, Barucand and Perse 1967 found connections between patients' consent and placebo responses. On the existence or not of placebo responders, see Wolf et al. 1957; Liberman 1967; Kaptchuk et al 2008.

20. On desire and motivation for health improvement, see, for example, Hyland, Whalley and Geraghty 2007; Price, Finniss and Benedetti 2008.

conditioned placebo effects (Benedetti et al. 2011, 345–346).[21] Although there might be a great variety of stimuli and different peripheral access points and pathways of signalling, the Central Nervous System seems to be involved in the behavioural conditioning. Therefore, regarding the neural pathways of the conditioned placebo responses, their formation and later recall seem to be localized in the insular cortex, while the visceral information enters the amygdala at the time of formation. Then 'behaviourally conditioned immune responses' are mediated by the ventromedial hypothalamic nucleus which constitutes 'the output pathway to the immune system' (Benedetti et al. 2011, 346; see, for example, Hucklebridge 2002, 348; Pacheco-Lopez et al. 2005, 2006; Daruna 2012, 110).

Although placebo responses are thought to be generated by unconscious processes of conditioning and associative learning, their inducement and effectiveness can further be reinforced by patients' expectations about the applied treatments.[22] The manipulation of expectations via verbal suggestions, for example, seems to affect the ways in which people experience sensory stimuli which trigger pain as well as their motor systems and central neural regulators of fatigue.[23] In particular, dopamine release in the ventral and dorsal striatum, after a placebo administration, and the subsequent neural changes in the subthalamic nucleus, substantia nigra pars reticulate and ventral anterior and anterior ventral lateral thalamus, which occur through cognitive learning and manipulation of expectations, can generate enhanced placebo responses which further may affect the sensory and motor systems of patients with Parkinson's disease

---

21. On the role of associative learning and behavioural conditioning in the activation of animals' immune systems, see Ader and Cohen 1975. On the activation of the human immune system, see Goebel et al. 2002, 2005, 2009. On the role of associative learning and conditioning in the activation of the endocrine system, see Lichko 1959; Alvarez-Buyalla and Carrasco-Zanini, 1960; Alvarez-Buyalla et al 1961; Woods et al, 1968, 1969, 1972; Woods 1972; Stockhorst et al 1999, 2000.
22. On the significance of expectations even during associative learning and conditioning, see, for example, Montgomery and Kirsch 1997.
23. The manipulation of expectations seems to affect placebo responses in Parkinson's disease, thus improving patients' motor performance; Pollo et al. 2002. Placebo effects seem to have similar impacts on sensory input and motor output of healthy individuals; Pollo, Carlino and Benedetti 2008, 347. Verbal communication and the manipulation of expectations seems to also mediate the nocebo effects; see Benedetti et al. 2003, 2007. For a review of current neurobiological models of placebo and nocebo effects, see Enck, Benedetti and Schedlowski 2008.

(Benedetti et al. 2011, 348; see further de la Fuente-Fernández et al. 2001, 2002b; Benedetti et al. 2004, 2011, 346–347).

Social learning seems to be even more powerful in the inducement of placebo responses than the manipulation of expectations through verbal communication. This learning is grounded in the observation or imitation of others' behaviours (see, for example, Henrich 2015, 124–126; Laland 2017, 52, 276–281). People who belong to the same social group may share common anticipations and expectations of future conditions. Social learning seems to generate placebo responses similar to those induced by associative learning and conditioning (e.g. Benedetti et al. 2011, 348; Bootzin and Caspi 2002; Siegel 2002; Colloca and Benedetti 2009).

Beyond the pan-human biological, neural, cognitive and psychological grounds of the placebo effect, there are significant cultural differences in responsiveness to placebo interventions (Moerman 2000, 2002; Humphrey 2005, 2; Diener et al. 2008). These variations could illuminate the way in which attitudes and dispositions toward doctors, medicine and body symbolism, shared by people of the Graeco-Roman world (see, for example, Harper 2017, ch. 3), might have generated placebo responses to Asclepius supplicants. In this perspective, the healing processes taking place at the Asclepius sanctuaries could base their efficacy not only on various treatments, but also on those cognitive and emotional features which allow humans to activate their own self-healing mechanisms.

Nicholas Humphrey's Theory of Placebo Effects

Nicholas Humphrey, in his chapter 'Great Expectations: The Evolutionary Psychology of Faith-Healing and the Placebo Effect' (2002), investigates the evolutionary origins of the placebo effect. His study illuminates the ways in which placebos activate the regular physiological processes of self-healing, without any external intervention beyond the implantation of particular ideas in the mind. According to his view, the human capacity for placebo responses constitutes a by-product of a more likely adaptive process which has developed to manage the available resources of human organisms enabling them to cope with illnesses, lesions and other threats of personal well-being (Humphrey 2002, 261).[24]

---

24. Arthur K. Shapiro and Elaine Shapiro were the first to emphasize the possible inherent features of placebo effects which developed through adaptation during evolution: 'Does

During their evolution, human beings have developed self-generated means of defence, like pain,[25] fatigue and fever,[26] against dangerous situations which can cause more serious damage to the organisms. These defensive mechanisms are not themselves biological malfunctions but appropriate adaptive responses expressed as symptoms which, by being unpleasant, alert humans to be more careful in the face of other more real threats, like bodily injuries, illnesses and diseases, and force them to seek rest and relief (Humphrey 2002, 264–266; cf. Nesse and Williams 1994, 1998). In addition, the immune system has developed to detect and recognize a wide range of pathogens (viruses, bacteria, parasites, fungi, etc.) which inflict the human organism causing diseases and to launch attacks against the infectious agents that it normally distinguishes from the healthy tissue.[27] The extent and intensity to which the defensive mechanisms and the immune system will be activated depends on the evaluation of the wider conditions under which an injury, a biological disruption or an infliction caused by a pathogen took place. This evaluation is a largely autonomous process and entails the appropriate management of the organism's internal resources for healthcare (Humphrey 2002, 262–264). In particular, the activation of the immune system is an extremely costly biological process which demands extensive amounts of energy and internal resources along with the assessment of the external conditions for executing an optimal response to the given situations (Humphrey 2002, 267; cf. Sheldon and Verhulst 1996; Owens and Wilson 1999; Muehlenbein et al. 2010).

Universal features of the physical and psychological environments determine the assessment of the costs and benefits of illness and recovery, and prompt people to activate more or less extensively their own self-healing

---

the ubiquity of the placebo effect throughout history suggest the possibility, popular but hardly testable today, or perhaps ever, that positive placebo effects are an inherited adaptive characteristic, conferring evolutionary advantages by reducing despondency, depression and hopelessness, and that allowed more people with the placebo trait to survive than those without it?' (Shapiro and Shapiro 1997b, 31).

25. On pain as a means of defence used by animals and humans to cope with health threats, see, for example, Nesse 1991; Broom 1998, 2001.

26. On fever as a product of natural choice that helps humans to counter infections, see, for example, Berlim and Abeche 2001; Styrt and Sugarman 1990; Kluger et al 1996.

27. There are cases in which the immune system turns against the organism itself and attacks healthy substances, organs and tissue, causing very serious autoimmune diseases and disorders (Humphrey 2002, 267). On the immune diseases, see, for example, Cotsapas and Hafler 2013.

mechanisms. In this view, the contexts which make people feel cheerful and safe (social acceptance, loved ones, familiar places, comforting rituals) are associated with more benefits from experiencing precautionary defences, fewer benefits from being ill, and lower costs of self-healing, allowing humans to deploy full-scale defensive and immune responses. On the other hand, settings that elicit feelings of anxiety, insecurity and loneliness (social rejection, foes, unknown places, ordeals) are related to lower benefits from intense precautionary defences, higher benefits from the symptoms of an illness and higher costs of self-healing urging people to retain powers and resources for later potential risks of survival and well-being (Humphrey 2002, 271). In short, as Humphrey (2005, 3) aptly points out, 'the brighter the prospects for a rapid recovery, the less to be gained from playing safe and remaining sick'.

Evolution has endowed humans – as well as other species – with the capacity to make appropriate use of their organism's resources, anticipating future events and thus their health mechanisms respond to a great extent predictably to universal environmental stimuli (Humphrey 2002, 271).[28] However, humans are not genetically evolved to anticipate every single situation that could have a direct impact on their health (Humphrey 2002, 272; cf. Henrich 2015, 54, 328–329; Laland 2017, 245–248). Instead, personal expectations are generated through complex higher order cognitive processing, including individuals' learning associations, reasoning and beliefs. People have particular representations and information which engender certain expectations about how things are going to be for them (Humphrey 2002, 272; cf. Shanks 2010). These expectations in turn induce hope or despair which are two sides of the same coin – both are forms of the emotional variable which allows humans to formulate respectively positive or negative anticipations about the future. Hope and despair, thus, constitute universal human emotions, designed to respond to external stimuli with the appropriate means of healthcare (Humphrey 2002, 272).

Placebos are treatments mainly based on hope, although the reason could be actually spurious, and placebo responses have developed as adaptive mechanisms of the human internal system of healthcare.[29] According

---

28. On the activation cost of the immune system under stressful conditions, see, for example, Svensson et al. 1998.
29. Humphrey refers to the research of one of his colleagues at the New School, Shlomo Breznitz (1999), who has explored how the inducement of certain expectations and hopes may affect individuals' experiences of anxiety, fatigue or pain tolerance.

to Humphrey (2002, 275; for further analysis see Humphrey 1995), there are three ways in which people can form a new belief that can further generate and sustain hope. The first way is *'personal experience'*. Patients who suffered from the same illness and received an effective treatment in the past, tend to believe that this experience can be repeated in the present. The interrelation of recovery to specific colours, sounds, labels, persons and so on, builds up learning associations which ascribe a certain effectiveness to otherwise elusive treatments (Humphrey 2002, 276).[30] These learning associations provide further the ground for the second way of believing and thereby hoping in recovery, that is, of *'rational argument'* which Humphrey (2002, 275) determines as the ability 'to reason your way to the belief by logical argument' (cf. Grünbaum 1981). Specific associations between treatments which have been proved to be effective and specific attributes of remedies, drugs and medical interventions, comprise the rational base of the former's effectiveness. In that case, 'active placebos' (injections, surgeries, etc.) usually give the sense of actual effective medical interventions to patients who believe that these kinds of methods are prerequisite to a cure. Similarly, the patients' involvement in the process of a cure can be rationalized as a requisite parameter of treatment and recovery (Humphrey 2002, 276; cf. Herrnstein 1962; Wickramasekera 1980). The third and perhaps most operative way in which patients can believe in and hope for recovery is the *assurance* that an *external authority* provides for them (Humphrey 2002, 275; cf. Kaptchuk 2002, 819–820). People who suffer from an illness can feel despair until somebody who is considered trustworthy and respectful assures them that their recovery is feasible, and is going to happen. In this case, people seem to need an external motivation in order to activate their own self-healing mechanisms, since they are not sufficiently self-reliant to believe what they themselves select to believe (Humphrey 2002, 275, 277–278).

In brief, according to Humphrey (2002, 257–258), the placebo effects can operate under four specific preconditions: (a) the patient should be aware that he or she receives or is going to receive a specific treatment;[31] (b) he or she believes that this treatment is effective; (c) his or her belief

---

30. On the significance of previous experiences and learning associations in the placebo effect, see, for example, Voudouris, Peck and Coleman 1985.
31. Placebo responses largely depend on patients' self-consciousness and awareness of treatment, while part of their attention turns to the wider context of the healing encounter; see, for example, Colloca and Benedetti 2006.

generates the expectation that, if he or she follows this treatment, he or she is going to feel better; (c) this expectation activates his or her capacity for self-healing, thus accelerating the desirable health outcome.[32]

Furthermore, the placebo treatments tend to be effective when they are applied to specific illnesses and inflicted bodily parts. This suggests that their outcomes are not simply the result of alterations of the patient's general moods and attitudes. Instead, it seems that the patient's expectations about the treatment's effectiveness on a certain illness 'must be being channelled into a relatively narrow and "appropriate" response' (Humphrey 2005, 2).

Taking into account these biological, cognitive and emotional features common to the human species as well as the specific historical, cultural and social contexts of the Graeco-Roman world, the following chapters apply theories of placebo effects on Asclepius' worshippers and investigate patients' interactions with themselves, their surroundings and the prospect of recovery and well-being.[33]

---

32. On the role of expectations in the effectiveness of medical treatments see, for example, Mitchell, Laurent and De Wit 1996.
33. A preliminary application of Humphrey's theory of the placebo effect on the Asclepius cult has been published in Panagiotidou 2016a.

Chapter 2

Forming Ideas about Asclepius and His Healing Power

The Asclepius cult became popular among people of the ancient Greek and Roman world for the divine healings that his supplicants were claimed to experience at his temples. His name is known since the age of Homer, who mentions him as a mortal doctor. However, his figure was radically transformed in ancient Greek mythology, which sketches out his gradual elevation from a mortal doctor to a god of healing. Asclepius developed into the supreme healing deity of Greek antiquity, and his name and figure as well as the associated mythical saga all promoted his mastery of medicine and interest in human needs.

In this chapter, I briefly review the ancient literary sources that preserve the major mythical sagas about Asclepius, his development into a divine healer and his relationship to human doctors. In particular, I begin from the first references in the Homer's *Iliad* and later in the *Homeric Hymn to Asklepios* and then present the mythical narratives about Asclepius written by Hesiod (*Cat.*), Pindar (*Pyth.* III), and Apollodorus (*Bibl.*) as well as some local variations of the Asclepius myths found in Pausanias' *Descriptio Graeciae* (*Descr. Graec.*). I then examine those representations and ideas in mythical narratives that would have made the stories about Asclepius particularly catching and memorable for people of that era, taking into account the theories of Stewart Guthrie (1992) and Pascal Boyer (2002) about the attractiveness of religious representations.

I also refer to the works collected in the *Corpus Hippocraticum* (*Hippocratic Corpus*)[1] that bears the name of Hippocrates, but contains about 60 treatises possibly written by more than one author in the long period from

---

1. The form of the collection as it is preserved today was printed by the Aldine press in Venice in 1526 CE and probably contains the compilation of texts collected by the scholars of the Alexandrian Library in the third century BCE; see further Nutton 2005, 60–64.

420–350 BCE to the first or second century CE. These works are thought to reflect the discussions about medicine and the role of doctors in the treatment of patients that took place among professional physicians over a long period and the ways in which people of that era would have perceived health and sickness and formed specific expectations about human physicians, divine healing and particularly Asclepius. At this point, I use the schema of medical pluralism suggested by Arthur Kleinman in order to trace the interaction and overlap between various ideas and attitudes toward human medicine, divine healing and other healing opportunities that existed in the wider cultural contexts of Greek antiquity. What I suggest is that the Asclepius cult developed into an attractive healing option for people of that era because it combined the ideas and expectations raised by both professional doctors and divine healers.

Asclepius: God and Doctor

The name Asclepius signifies a propitious and kind nature and the desire to serve human well-being. According to ancient sources the name was a compound containing the word ἤπιος (-epios), which means mild. Indeed, there seems to be a consensus among ancient authors that mildness was a major feature of the god (Plut. *X orat.* VIII, 845B = T. 266;[2] Porph. *Quest. Home.* a, 68 = T. 269; Schol. Hom. *Il.* IV, 195 = T. 270; Schol. Lycophr. *Ad Alexandram*, 1054 = T. 271; Eust. *Il.* IV, 202 = T. 272; *Etym. Gudianum, s.v.* Ἀσκληπιός = T. 274; *Etym. Magn. s.v.* Ἀσκελές = T. 275; Sudas s.v. Ἀσκληπιάδης = T. 276).[3] Although there is less agreement on the meaning of (Ascl-), it is apparent that Asclepius was considered to be the benevolent deity who soothed and healed the suffering and helped defer death. '"Asclepius" was named from his healing softly, and putting off the stiffness that comes about at death' (Cornutus, *Theol.* Cp. 33, trans. Boys-Stones 2018).

His smooth hands soothed the pains of the sick, and made both their limbs and whole body soft (*Etym. Gudianum, s.v.* Ἀσκληπιός). He was the one who could lessen the harshness of disease (*Etym. Magn. s.v.* Ἀσκελές).

---

2. The citations (T.) used by Edelstein and Edelstein (1998) for the ancient *testimonia* about Asclepius are included in the references throughout the text.
3. On the etymology of the name 'Asclepius', see, for example, Edelstein and Edelstein 1998, v. II, 80–3; Hart 2000, 5; Riethmüller 2005, v. I, 33–54; Beekes 2009, 151; Błaśkiewicz 2014, 57.

The mythical saga developed around the figure of Asclepius also underlined his healing abilities (cf. Hes. *Cat.* fr. 123 = T. 22; Pind. *Pyth.* III, 1–58 = T. 1; Apollod. *Bibl.* III, 10, 3, 5–4, 1 = T. 3; Hom. *Hymn Ascl.* XVI, 1–5 = T. 31; Paus. *Descr. Graec.* II, 26, 3–5, 7, VIII, 25, 11 = T. 7, 17). The first references to his name are found in the *Iliad*. Homer presents him as the father of two heroes-doctors of the Trojan War, Machaon and Podalirius, heads of the army of Trikka, Itheme and Oechalia (see Nutton 2005, 38). Although his status as the king of these regions is only indirectly implied, and he is briefly mentioned as the father of these heroes, Homer speaks of Asclepius' medical skills. The epic poet characterizes him as a 'blameless physician' (ἀμύμονος ἰητῆρος; see Hom. *Il.* IV, 194, XI, 504–520, 518 = T. 165; T. 164) who had received remedies and simples from the centaur Chiron (Hom. *Il.* XI, 219 = T. 50). These early poetic references to Asclepius imply that stories about both his figure and medical virtue were already known from the second half of the eighth century BCE (Panagiotidou 2016b).[4]

Over time, more detailed myths, narrating the origins, birth, life and death of Asclepius as well as his training as a physician, were formulated, and determined his position in both the human and the divine realms. In the *Catalogue of Women* (*Gynaikôn Katálogos* fr. 123 = T. 22), which was composed in the early sixth century BCE and was attributed to Hesiod, Apollo is presented as the father of Asclepius who had the child either with Arsinoë, the daughter of Leucippus from Messene, or with Coronis, the daughter of Phlegyas from Thessaly (Edelstein and Edelstein 1998, v. II, 24). Regarding Coronis, Hesiod briefly mentions that she married a mortal man, named Ischys, the son of Elatus, when Apollo was absent in Pytho and was informed about her marriage by a raven.

This mythical version which presented Coronis as the mother of Asclepius is more extensively preserved in the third of the *Pythiae Odes* (*Pyth.* III, 1–58 = T. 1) composed by Pindar in the first half of the fifth century BCE. In this narrative, Apollo became intimate with Coronis who got pregnant. But while she was carrying the god's baby, she was involved in a relationship with Ischys. A raven brought the message of Coronis' infidelity to Apollo who in high rage changed the bird's colour from white to black and asked his sister, Artemis, to kill the woman. But while Coronis

---

4. On the various mythical sagas about Asclepius see, for example, Kerényi 1959, 87–99; Meier 1967, 19–39; Martin and Metzger 1992, 74–75, 84; Edelstein and Edelstein 1998, v. II, 24–53, 76; Hart 2000, 7–10; Nutton 2005, 104; Riethmüller 2005, v. I, 33–54; Mattern 2013, 26; Błaśkiewicz 2014, 57–59; Steger 2018, 37–63.

was on fire, Apollo decided to save his son. Thus, he passed through the fire which opened a path for him and detached the baby from his mother's womb. Then he delivered Asclepius to the Magnesian centaur Chiron who took care of and raised the child. Under the tutelage of Chiron, Asclepius was taught the art of healing and was trained to become a physician of high competence who cured human illnesses and diseases and relieved suffering. His healing abilities became so great that he surpassed human limits by resurrecting people from death. Such a deed was considered to be impious by Zeus, who therefore punished Asclepius with death by striking him with a thunderbolt (Panagiotidou 2016b).[5]

The *Bibliotheca* (*Bibl*. III, 10, 3, 5–4, 1 = T. 3), a compilation of myths and legends, that was in all probability composed in the first or second century CE and is attributed to Pseudo-Apollodorus, preserves the mythical saga of Asclepius. This testimony mentions Arsinoë as the mother of Asclepius, while citing the myth of Coronis in more detail. The story agrees with the myth delivered by Pindar but proceeds beyond the slaughtering of Asclepius by Zeus. Being trained by Chiron, Asclepius became a great physician and surgeon whose skills overpassed the limits of the human medical art. The extraordinary healing powers of Asclepius moved him to cure people who were destined to die using the blood of Gorgon, which Athena had given to him. But by saving people from dying and reviving the dead, he threatened the predominance of the gods in the realms of the human life and death. Zeus worried that the opportunity provided by Asclepius to mortals to transcend their mortality would lead them to impiety and disrespect of the gods. Thus, he struck Asclepius by his thunderbolt and killed him. Appollo was infuriated by his son's slaughter and seeking revenge, he killed Cyclopes, Brontes, Steropes and Arges, who had manufactured Zeus' thunderbolts. In turn, Zeus being enraged threw Apollo into Tartarus. Later, the mother of Apollo, Leto, managed to convince Zeus to change his mind, and thus Apollo was withdrawn from Tartarus but was impelled to

---

5. The main events of the mythical saga, although with slight variations, were delivered by different sources, indicating that the story was quite known in Greek antiquity. Ferecydes (Schol. in Pind., *Ad Pythias*, III, 59 = T. 24), for instance, talks about the raven, but argues that Artemis slew Coronis along with many other women, while Apollo killed Ischys himself. Philodemus (*Piet*. 17 = T. 106) mentions the names of Pindar, Pherecydes, Panyassis, Andron, Acusilaus, Eyripides, Telestes and the author of Naupactia who also confirmed Hesiod in his claim that Zeus killed Asclepius. Ovid in his *Metamorphoses* (II, 542–648 = T. 2), written in the first century AD, tells a story very similar to that preserved by Pindar.

serve Admetus, son of Pheres, as a thrall for a year.[6] Regarding Asclepius, many ancient sources mention his deification after his murder by Zeus because of his unique medical competence and services to humankind.[7]

Despite the secondary variations, the main features and protagonists of the mythical story of Asclepius comprise commonplace highlighting crucial components of the beliefs developed around his figure. Thus, in all mythical versions, Asclepius is presented as the son of Apollo belonging to the divine lineage of the Olympian gods. The divine healing powers of his father, who was the main Olympian god with a special concern for human health, as well as his training by centaur Chiron, who was known as the doctor who invented herbal medicine and the first to use drugs to cure illnesses, gave grounds for the extraordinary healing powers and medical competence of Asclepius who became the kindest provider and guarantor of good health (Schol. in Pind., *Ad Pythias* III, 102b = T. 54).

In addition, his mortal parentage on the side of his mother justified his relationship with the human world and his concerns in people's health and well-being (Panagiotidou 2016b). Therefore, the semiotics attributed to Asclepius' name and the myths about him imply the kinds of attitudes and feelings people shared towards him. His cult offered hope to patients suffering from illnesses and diseases, and they came to the sanctuaries to find relief from their ailments and a route to recovery.

---

6. The punishment of Apollo by Zeus because the former killed the Cyclopes is a commonplace in the ancient sources that deliver the myth of Asclepius; see Hes., Fr. 125 = T. 105; Philodemus, *Piet*. 17 = T. 106; Eur. *Alc*. 1–7 = T. 107; Schol. in Eurip. *Alc*. 1 = T. 108; Schol. in Lucianum, *Jovem Confut*. 8 = T. 109; Schol. in Ap. Rhod. *Argon*. IV, 611–617 = T. 110; Serv. *Comm. in Aen*. VI, 398 = T. 111; Origen, *C. Cels*. III, 23 = T. 112; Ambrosius, *De Virgin*. III, 176, 7 = T. 113; Firm. Mat. *Err. prof. rel*. XII, 8 = T. 114; Heraclitus, *Incredibil*. XXVI = T. 115 (cf. Wickkiser 2008, 44–50).

7. Min. Fel. *Oct*. XXIII = T. 236; Hyg. *Fab*., CCLI, 2, CCXXIV = T. 237, 238; Cic., *Nat. D*. II, 24, 62 = T. 239; Cic. *Leg*. II, 8, 19; Cic. *Nat. D*. III, 18, 45 = T. 252; Porph. *Ep. ad Marc*. 7 = T. 241; Origen, *Jer. Hom*. V, 3 = T. 242; Origen, *C. Cels*. III, 22 = T. 249; Xen. *Cyn*. I, 6 = T. 243; Celsus, *Med. Prooem*. 2; Gal. *Protr*. 9, 22; Athenagoras, *Leg*. 30, 1–2 = T. 246; Georg. Hamart. *Chron*. I, 54 = T. 247; August. *De civ. D*. IV, 27, VIII, 5 = T. 248, 253; Lactant. *Div. inst*. I, 15, 26, I, 19, 3–4 = T. 251, 250; Apul. *De Deo Soc*. XV, 153 = T. 254; Paus. *Descr. Graec*. II, 26, 10 = T. 255; Eust. *Il*. XI, 517–518 = T. 256.

Divine Nascence, Anthropomorphism and the Perception of Asclepius as a Superhuman Healer

The mythical saga presented Asclepius as a mortal doctor of extraordinary competence who was deified by Zeus because of his unique skills and accomplishments. As already mentioned, his divine nascence from the side of his father, Apollo, ranked him in the kin of the Olympian gods and at some extent grounded his superhuman powers. Particularly, the anthropomorphic perception of gods and deities in Greek antiquity seems to have mediated the development of the religious ideas about Asclepius and his divine nature.[8]

Anthropomorphism generally consists in the attribution of human-like physical, biological and psychological qualities to non-human agents. According to Guthrie (1992), the anthropomorphic perception of various components of the world constitutes an adaptive interpretative response to potential threats that might derive from the presence and activity of other human or non-human live agents in people's surroundings. Humans have developed the tendency to initially interpret perceivable entities and their traces in space in anthropomorphic terms, since such interpretation increases the possibilities of survival in case that a potential threat deriving from other agents' activity actually exists. The anthropomorphic perception and interpretation of the world is largely promoted by various religious traditions that develop ideas about superhuman agents who interact with the human world and communicate with humans in multiple ways (Guthrie 1992, 178).

Boyer (2002) has further explored the major components found in the majority of the religious ideas about superhuman agents across the world that make these ideas particularly memorable and attractive to people in different times and places. According to his theoretical premises, humans continually perceive and interpret their surroundings classifying any perceptible entity they encounter in one of five major ontological categories (i.e. those of persons, animals, plants, tools and natural objects). Each of these categories is associated with a certain set of intuitive expectations pertaining to the biological, psychological and physical domains. These expectations are unconsciously triggered by and attributed to every perceptible entity.

---

8. A preliminary presentation of the major ideas of this section was originally published in Panagiotidou 2016b.

Religious agents are generally within the major ontological categories of the perceivable world and activate the relevant intuitive expectations. What makes these agents particularly salient and attention-grabbing, however, is some slight violation of the domain-specific expectations that their classification in a specific ontological category induces. According to Boyer's, this violation should be minimal, since it should not demand extensive cognitive efforts to be processed, kept in memory and recalled, and simultaneously should not demolish people's overall perception of reality and worldview. This minimal violation, which balances between the rational and the irrational, grabs the attention, causes surprise and provokes curiosity, thus facilitating the memorability and transmission of the relevant ideas. In particular, the research of Michaela Porubanova-Norquist and her colleagues (2013, 2014) has shown that ideas which violate intuitive expectations triggered by the ontological category of persons tend to be more attention-grabbing and memorable than violations of expectations pertaining to the other ontological categories.[9]

Anthropomorphic perception seems to lie at the heart of the ancient Greek religion.[10] The gods and deities of Greek antiquity were imagined as human-like agents who displayed the major physical, biological and psychological qualities pertaining to the ontological category of persons.[11] Thus, they were represented as physically and anatomically similar to humans, males and females with unique outward appearances and bodily characteristics.[12] They had also certain biological needs similar to those inherent to humans. They ate and drank, slept and woke up, made love

---

9. See, however, the critical discussion of research results on minimally counterintuitive ideas in Purzycki and Willard 2016, with peer commentaries.

10. I mainly refer to the popular religious ideas as they were expressed in mythical sagas and not to the philosophical and theological discussions about the gods and divinity which took place already in antiquity. Anthropomorphic perception would have grounded the ways in which people of the ancient Greek world would have conceived and spontaneously reasoned about superhuman agents and divine interventions in their ordinary lives. On the academic debates regarding anthropomorphism in ancient Greek religion, see, for example, Webster 1954; Vernant 1991; Bremmer 1994, 12; Henrichs 2010, 32–35; Versnel 2011, 266, 317, 382–383; Kindt 2012, 42–43.

11. As Versnel (2011, 317) aptly points out, 'in everyday religious practice individual Greek gods were practically never conceived of as powers, let alone as cultural products, but were in the first place envisaged as persons with individual characters and personalities' (see also Versnel 2011, 382–383; cf. Guthrie 1992, 186).

12. On the incorporation of the ancient Greek gods in human bodies, see Vernant 1991; Osborne 2011, 185–215; Kindt 2012, 43–47, 157–161.

and gave birth to offspring (see, for example, Vernant 1991, 34–36). They also shared common psychological traits with humans. They had feelings and emotions. They felt love and hate, envy and sympathy, joy and sorrow, happiness and sadness. They had further unique mentalities and personalities, developed personal preferences and attitudes, and had different fields of expertise.[13] They were connected with each other through social relationships and developed social networks composed of relatives, friends and acquaintances from both the divine and the human realm. Thus, they were much human-like agents with one major difference: they did not face the prospect of death, and their immortality was in great contrast to the inevitable mortality of the human species (see, for example, Hom. *Il.* V, 441–442; Hes. *Theog.* 938–942, 949, 954–955; cf. Dodds 1965, 74; Jost 1992, 18; Bremmer 1994, 12; Versnel 2011, 391–392). I suggest that this was the minimal violation of one of the intuitive biological expectations ascribed to humans which would have made the Greek deities particularly interesting and attention-attractive figures.

In this conceptual context, the mythical saga presented Asclepius as an originally mortal man who was the offspring of a masculine god and a feminine human. He was trained in the art of medicine and over time became a great physician, following more or less the career of mortal doctors. The anthropomorphic appearance and character of Asclepius as a healer and physician, indicated by the earliest references to him and highlighted by the mythical stories about his origins and deeds, was further supported and clearly manifested by visual imagery. He was depicted as a mature bearded man clothed with a himation,[14] holding a wooden staff with a serpent entwined around it – the so-called *caduceus,* which became

---

13. Ares, for instance, was the god of war, Artemis the goddess of the hunt, Athena the goddess of arts and wisdom, Demeter the goddess of agriculture and harvest and so on.

14. Historians suggested that some earlier representations of a young naked man who holds a *caduceus* display Asclepius. They interpreted the youthfulness of his image as a symbol of medical treatment and rejuvenation of a suffering body. In the fifth century BCE the Greek sculptor Calamis represented gods as young men (e.g. Paus. *Descr. Graec.* II, 10, 3 = T. 649). Some ancient scholars, like Cicero (*Nat. D.* III, 34, 83 = T. 683), found it difficult to accept the representations of Apollo as a youth, while his son was a middle-aged man. Warwick Wroth (1882) argues that the depictions of a young man who holds a staff with a serpent entwined represent Apollo instead of Asclepius. In any case, the image of the mature bearded man with *caduceus* prevailed as the typical representation of Asclepius after the fourth century BCE; on the interpretations of 'Asclepius adolescent', see Hart 2000, 22–26.

the symbol of medicine.[15] His figure resembled the stereotypical representations of doctors and was presumably easily recognizable by contemporaries.[16] His expression was calm and kind, while his eyes did not focus on a specific point, but gazed into the distance (Edelstein and Edelstein 1998, v. II, 218–225). Such imagery was consistent with a benevolent nature, wishing to save humankind from suffering (Figure 1).

Regarding his social status, Asclepius was related genealogically to the Olympian gods. However, he was at the periphery of the social network comprised by the gods who resided atop Mount Olympus and were direct descendants of Cronus and Rhea, or of Zeus,[17] who along with his brothers and sisters beat the Titans. However, as Asclepius grew up and came of age, another social network developed around him which shared a common concern in human health and specific healing abilities. Thus, Asclepius was presented to have married the daughter of Hercules, Epione,[18] who represented 'the alleviation of troubles through the agency of soothing simples' (Cornutus, *Theol.* Cp. 33 = T. 6). In addition to the Homeric doctors, Machaon and Podalirius, Asclepius and Epione had offspring that acquired certain medical powers and occasionally accompanied their father in the practice of medicine. The most permanent partner of Asclepius in temple medicine was his daughter Hygeia – the personification of Health.[19]

---

15. On *caduceus*, see, for example, Cilliers and Retief 2005, 191–196; Rillo 2008, 389–393; Nayernouri 2010, 61–68; Antoniou et al. 2011.

16. A fragmentary relief dated in the late sixth or early fifth century BCE is the first preserved representation of the stereotypical image of doctors. It represents a bearded, seated man who holds a walking staff and faces another younger, possibly male figure not well-preserved. Cupping instruments, which were used as therapeutic tools by physicians, are included in the representation. Another representation is preserved on a marble disk dated in the late sixth century. Although the painting is not so well-preserved, it represents a doctor in the same posture, and bears the inscription: ΜΝΗΜΑ ΤΟΔ ΑΙΝΕΟ ΣΟΦΙΑΣ ΙΑΤΡΟ ΑΡΙΣΤΟ ('This is a memorial of the skill of Aineas, best of doctors', trans. Wickkiser 2008, 18); on the first relief, see Wickkiser 2008, 17–18 and particularly Berger 1970, 30–33, who dates it around 480 BCE, and Nutton 1992, 20, who dates it in the sixth century; on the marble disk, see Marshall 1909, 154; Berger 1970, 155–18l; Samama 2003, no 001; Wickkiser 2008, 18.

17. Dionysus was the only Olympian god who was the son of Zeus and of a mortal woman, Semele, princess of Thebes.

18. Her name contained the second compound of Asclepius' name '-epios' ('mild').

19. In some cases, Hygeia is presented as being the wife of Asclepius (see, for example, *Hymn. Orph.* LXVII = T. 601); on Hygeia see Hart 2000, 29–31; Beumer 2016; on the relation between Hygeia and Asclepius, see Compton 2002, 329; Renberg 2017, 117–118.

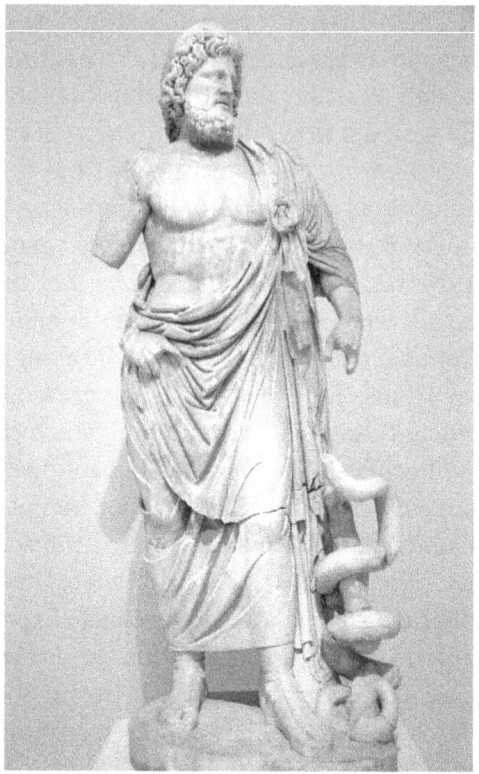

Figure 1 Statue of Asclepius from the *asclepieion* of Epidaurus, National Archaeological Museum of Athens.

Source: Carole Raddato from Frankfurt, Germany, CC BY-SA 2.0, https://creativecommons.org/licenses/by-sa/2.0, via Wikimedia Commons

Panacea,[20] who, it was believed, had a 'universal remedy' and cured every illness and disease; Iaso,[21] who represented the healing process; Aceso,[22] who signified recovery; and Aegle, who possibly implied the splendor of the healthy human body or the glory of the medical profession (Greenhill 1867, 27), were also considered to be the Asclepius' daughters personifying

---

20. The doctors who took the Hippocratic Oath swore by Apollo, Asclepius, Hygeia and Panacea (Hippoc. *Ius Iur.* 1= T. 337; Lloyd 1979, 43; Hart 2000, 31).
21. The name Iaso etymologically derives from the ancient Greek verb *iasthai* (ἰᾶσθαι) which means 'to heal' (Schol. Ar. *Plut.* 701 = T. 285).
22. The name of Aceso comes for the ancient Greek verb *akeesthai* (ἀκέεσθαι) which means 'to heal and recover'.

aspects of their father's medical art (*IG* II(2), 4962 = T. 515; Anon. *Pae. Erythr. Ascl.* = T. 592; Plin. *H.N.* XXXV, 11 (40), 137 = T. 665; Schol. in Ar. *Plut.* 639 = T. 278; see Leventi 2003, 46–54; Stafford 2005, 130–132; Kranz 2010, 56–58). In the Roman era, another secondary deity, Telesphoros ('the accomplisher'), who was associated with sleep, good health, and magical treatments, was added in the medical family as a son of Asclepius (*IG* III, 1, 1159 = T. 287; Dam. *Dubit. Solut.* 245 = T. 313; Hart 2000, 33; Stafford 2005, 130–132).

Therefore, in both mythical stories and visual representations Asclepius was a fully anthropomorphized figure who would have been classified in the ontological category of persons, thus triggering the full range of intuitive expectations induced by this category. The minimal violation, in Boyer's terms (2002), which would have made his figure particularly interesting and memorable for people of Greek antiquity is his extraordinary accomplishments. By resurrecting the dead, Asclepius pushed his medical art beyond the limits of human abilities and transgressed the borders of the divine realm. Only the gods were immortals and were not under the dominance of Hades. By winning over death, Asclepius violated the intuitive expectations of what humans can accomplish, and, according to Boyer's theory (2002), such an idea would have been enough to grab people's attention and to be recalled and transmitted.

The deification of Asclepius by Zeus is presented in the myths as following upon the superhuman deeds he performed as a mortal doctor. Since immortality was considered to be the major counterintuitive concept ascribed to the ancient Greek gods, its attribution to Asclepius derived from his elevation to the rank of deities which would have comprised a specific cultural category in the ancient Greek worldview (see Panagiotidou 2016b).

Asclepius: An Anthropomorphized Superhuman Physician and His Mortal Counterparts

By resurrecting the dead, Asclepius violated not only the intuitive expectations shared by humans about their mortal nature, but also the common cultural expectations that people of the ancient Greek world had about healing gods, medicine and the human doctors.

In the first place, after his deification, Asclepius shared with other ancient Greek gods and deities the superhuman power to heal human illnesses and diseases. Anatomical votive offerings that were found mainly on the island of Crete,[23] and dated back in the Bronze Age, indicate that people very early turned to divine help when they were confronted by health issues (see Van Straten 1981, 105-151, esp. 146; Georgoulaki 1997, 198-202; Holmes 2008, 101; Wickkiser 2008, 33; Panagiotidou 2016a, 81). At least from the Homeric Age, the gods were widely considered to be the origins of the human illnesses and diseases as well as those who could bring recovery, and people used to ask for their aid.[24] Among the Olympian gods, Apollo was mainly associated with human health and well-being and appeared to perform miraculous healings.[25]

Along with the superhuman powers of Asclepius that derived from his deification and his elevation to the status of a god, the son of Apollo displayed some unique features which differentiated him from his divine colleagues, and attributed to him superior medical abilities and healing competence. The other deities appeared to have innate healing powers acquired without previous training. Their ability to heal was one of their

---

23. On the votive offerings which represented bodily limbs and have been found on the Cretan Peak sanctuaries, see, for example, Peatfield 1990; Nowicki 1994; Jones 1999; Morris 2009; Morris and Peatfield 2014.

24. For instance, in the *Iliad* (I, 43-67), Apollo is represented as the one who sent the plague to the Greek camp and the one to whom the Greeks offered sacrifices asking for the elimination of the disease. On the divine origins and moral connotations of epidemic diseases that inflicted entire communities, see, for example, Parker 1983, 207-256; Gorrini 2005. Athena, Leto and Artemis appear along with Apollo to heal the wounds of their favoured heroes (Hom. *Il.* V, 114-122, 445-448, XVI, 508-529). Olympian gods had also their divine physician, Paieon, who cured their wounds using specific medical methods (*Il.* V, 363-415, 899). In the *Odyssey* (VI, 365), the gods appear to cure the indefinable illness of a man who lay 'in sickness, bearing grievous pains' (see Nutton 2005, 38-39; Wickkiser 2008, 34).

25. The association of Apollo with the domain of human health is indicated by the epithets which were ascribed to his name. In the regions of Asia Minor and the Black Sea, he was called Apollo Iatros (doctor) from the sixth century BCE. When the Romans evoked his divine intervention in order to be saved from a plague that had afflicted their city in the mid-fifth century BCE, they attributed to Apollo the epithet Medicus; see Ehrhardt 1989; Burkert 1994, 49-60; Hart 2000, 19; Nutton 2005, 107; Wickkiser 2008, 50-51; Graf 2009, 65-83; Ustinova 2009; Petridou 2016, 175-176. Beyond Apollo, other Olympian gods were involved in the domain of human health, and their cults acquired certain healing aspects in different regions. Thus, for instance, the anatomical votive offerings found at the sanctuaries of Artemis at Ephesus and at Lousoi in Arkadia indicate a healing aspect of her local cult (Wickkiser 2008, 34; Petridou 2014, 291-292). The association of Hera with the Babylonian healing deity Gula of Isin – a connection evident at the former's sanctuary on Samos – indicates that her cult had an obvious healing dimension (Wickkiser 2008, 34; Steger 2018, 18-19; on the cult of Gula, see Avalos 1995, 99-231; Böck 2014).

multiple supernatural powers, which enabled them to intervene in people's lives, to predict or even predetermine the future, and to affect human affairs. Thus, when the gods performed cures, they acted as more than mere physicians. Their treatments were often inexplicable, and far from the medical techniques used by mortal doctors. Asclepius, on the other hand, was recognized as a divine healer *par excellence*. Contrary to other deities,[26] his healing abilities were not among his inherent superhuman powers. He developed his medical skills through training. He continually studied developments in the medical art, and used the most advanced medical techniques and treatments in order to cure human illnesses and diseases (see Wickkiser 2008, 50-51; cf. Burkert 1985, 214-215).

Asclepius' medical expertise ranked him in the same class as human doctors, with whom he shared the same goal – the healing of ill people. Doctors quite early comprised a specific professional category, a development that is testified already in the Bronze Age.[27] Specific training and medical knowledge in treating mainly battle wounds[28] differentiated the Homeric doctors from other heroes who shared elementary first aid knowledge (e.g. Hom. *Il*. IV, 193-218, V, 902-904, IX, 804-848; see Wickkiser 2008, 12-14). At least from the sixth century BCE, human doctors were considered to be of high esteem, and there was a demand for their services in cities as the position of public doctors implies.[29]

---

26. In addition to deities, some heroes were also popular for their healing skills, and performed cures at their sanctuaries (Ferguson 2003, 222-223). The Athenian healing heroes are better documented; for example, Amphiaraos (e.g. Petrakos 1968, 1997; Schachter 1981, v. I, 19-26), Amynos (e.g. Purday 1987, 69-102); Heros Iatros (e.g. Usener 1896, 149-153; Rohde 1925, 133, 150-151; Kerényi 1945); see further Kearns 1989; Verbanck-Piérard 2000; Gorrini 2001, 2005; Vikela 2006; Wickkiser 2008, 51-52; Petridou 2014, 292.

27. For example, the word *i-ja-te*, which is considered to be a forerunner of the Greek word ἰατρός (doctor), first appeared on a tablet as well as in a Minoan inscription dated around 1550 BCE (see Wickkiser 2008, 10-11; see further Arnott 1996, 266, 2004, 157); on medical experts in the Bronze Age, see Laskaris 1999, 1-2, 2002, 32-39.

28. On treatments of battle wounds in Homeric poems and the pre-Hippocratic era, see, for example, Salazar 2000, 126-158; Santos 2000; Sahlas 2001.

29. A demand for doctors' services along with the public services offered by other professionals like prophets, builders and poets is already implied in *Odyssey* (17, 382-386): 'Who pray, of himself ever seeks out and bids a stranger from abroad, unless it be one of those that are masters of some public craft, a prophet, or a healer of ills, or a builder, aye, or a divine minstrel, who gives delight with his song? For these men are bidden all over the boundless earth' (trans. Murray 1919). At least from the late fifth century, some Greek cities organized annual competitions for filling the positions of public doctors; Wickkiser 2008, 16, 18-21; on public doctors, see, for example, Cohn-Haft 1956; Nutton 1977; Pleket

Upon the emergence of the Asclepius cult, human doctors were interested in establishing an affinity with the divine physician. From the fifth century BCE and particularly after the birth of Hippocrates on Kos (c. 460) and the establishment of his medical school at his motherland, Hippocratic doctors claimed their descent from Asclepius, and the term *Asclepiades* was used to underline this kinship.[30] Claiming their common divine origins, the doctors formed a kind of fraternity or even kinship in which the medical art tended to be transmitted from one generation to the next (see Burkert 1992, 44). This relationship among physicians was testified by the common oath they pledged to Asclepius. The *Hippocratic Oath*, which probably originated in the fifth century BCE, constituted a bond of commitments that doctors should uphold as long as they practised their profession (Lloyd 1979, 41; Burkert 1992, 44; Wickkiser 2008, 54; Mattern 2013, 26; Jouanna 2012, 113; Israelowich 2015, 112).[31]

The relation between Asclepius and his human disciples was enhanced over time and was manifested through the typical signs of medical art often borne on the medical kits and rings – the *caduceus* and the image of the divine physician (Wickkiser 2008, 57; Mikalson 2010, 223–224). Furthermore, evidence from the fourth century BCE indicates that doctors used to offer sacrifices to Asclepius, and to dedicate offerings to his sanctuaries.[32] In the first century BCE, various mythical narratives

---

1983; Jouanna 1999, 77–78; Chamoux 2003, 190–191; Israelowich 2015, 13–14, 42, 131–132; on professional doctors in Rome, see Israelowich 2014, 457–458, 2015, 12–29, 130.

30. For example, Plato in *Protagoras* (311 b–c) and in *Phaidrus* (270 c–d) refers to Hippocrates as a member of the family of Asclepiades. For the term 'Asclepiades' and the discussion whether it refers to the blood relatives of Asclepius, to the priests of the *asclepieia* or to all doctors, see Sherwin-White 1978, 262–263, 266–270; Smith 1990, 9–18; Edelstein and Edelstein 1998, v. II, 12–15, 54–63; Jouanna 1999, 10–12, 2012, 113–118; Wickkiser 2008, 54; Mattern 2013, 26. In Plato's *Symposium* (186c–e), possibly written in the early fourth century, but reflecting ideas already established by the previous century, the doctor Eryximachos presents Asclepius as the ancestor of physicians and founder of medicine: 'Now the most hostile are the most opposite, such as hot and cold, bitter and sweet, moist and dry, and the like. And my ancestor, Asclepius, knowing how to implant friendship and accord in these elements, was the creator of our art, as our friends the poets here tell us, and I believe them' (trans. Jowett 1956). The term 'Asclepiades' is also found in, e.g. Thgn. *Eleg*. 432–434 = T. 219, Eur. *Alc*. 965–971 = T. 220; Gal. *Intro. Cp*. 2 [XIV, p. 676K.] = T. 221; see also T. 222–231.

31. For a different dating of the *Hippocratic Oath*, see Edelstein 1943.

32. Inventory lists from the *asclepieia* in Athens (*IG* II(2), 1533.34, 86–87, 116, 1534A.84a, 1534B. 155, 161), Piraeus (*IG* II(2), 47.8–9, 11, 16–19) and Delos (*ID* 1414.9, 1416A II. 9–10) include various medical tools and implements that physicians probably devoted to their

related Hippocrates to Asclepius. A collection of letters (*Epistulae*), the *Pseudepigrapha*, ascribed to Hippocrates, presented the latter as a descendent of Asclepius. Asclepius once appeared to Hippocrates in a dream, and helped him cure a difficult condition (Hippoc. *Ep.* 2, 10, 17, 20; on the dream see *Ep.* 15). A mosaic, dated in the second or third century CE, probably displays Hippocrates welcoming Asclepius as he arrives at Kos by ship.[33] This depiction indicates that Hippocrates and the medical profession had already flourished there before Asclepius came to the island. Later ancient sources reversed the sequence of events and presented Hippocrates to have drawn his medical knowledge from the healing inscriptions of the Koan asclepieion. Strabo argued that Hippocrates based some of his treatments on the narrative inscriptions from the Koan asclepieion (Longrigg 1998, 48; Wickkiser 2008, 55; Israelowich 2015, 51): 'And it is said that the dietetics practised by Hippocrates were derived mostly from the cures recorded on the votive tablets there' (Strabo, *Geog.* XIV, 2, 19 = T. 794, trans. Jones 1924).

Meanwhile, Pliny, quoting Varro, presented Hippocrates copying the treatments written on the Koan votive inscriptions and, after the god's sanctuary was burned, establishing the clinical branch of medical practice using Asclepian therapeutic methods (Smith 1990, 11; Longrigg 1998, 48; Wickkiser 2008, 55; Israelowich 2015, 51): 'Hippocrates, it is said, copied out these prescriptions, and, as our fellow-countryman Varro will have it, after burning the temple to the ground, instituted that branch of medical practice which is known as "Clinics"' (Plin. *H.N.* 29, 2, trans. Bostock and Riley 1855).

However, archaeological excavations testify to the first story, according to which the Hippocratic medical school was established before the construction of the Asclepius sanctuary on Kos (Longrigg 1998, 48). The connection between the two supreme doctors was further promoted by coins minted on Kos that bore Hippocrates' head on one side and Asclepius' staff

---

patron god (Wickkiser 2008, 54–55; on the Athenian inventories, see Aleshire 1989; on the Delian inventories, see Hamilton 2000, 183–186, 190–191). An Athenian inscription (*IG* II(2), 772, 9–13 = T. 552) dated to the middle of the third century BCE records that it was 'traditional for public doctors to sacrifice to Asklepios and Hygieia twice a year both on behalf of themselves and the patients that each of them treated, for good fortune' (trans. Byrne, available at www.atticinscriptions.com/inscription/IGII2/772); on the inscription, see Samama 2003, no. 011; Nutton 2005, 111; Wickkiser 2008, 55; Israelowich 2015, 46.

33. On the mosaic, see Sherwin-White 1978, 275; Jouanna 1999, 5; Wickkiser 2008, 55.

with the serpent entwined on the other (Wickkiser 2008, 55; see further Sherwin-White 1978, 275).

In the Roman era, more doctors emphasized their associations with Asclepius.[34] In Athens, the doctors, who held the office of *zakoros*,[35] oversaw the daily rituals at the *asclepieion* on the Acropolis (Aleshire 1989, 59, 74, 87–88; Wickkiser 2008, 56, 2009; Lefantzis and Jensen 2009; Papaefthymiou 2009; Israelowich 2015, 66). In Ephesus, doctors offered annual sacrifices, and held the Great Festival of Asclepius, during which contests in medicine and surgery took place (Nutton 2005, 211, 281). In the first century CE, C. Stertinius Xenophon, the Koan doctor of the emperor Claudius, dedicated effusive offerings to the *asclepieion* of his motherland.[36] He also served as a priest of Asclepius, while coins were minted bearing his image according to the pattern of those depicting Hippocrates (Nutton 2005, 255–256; Wickkiser 2008, 55–56; Israelowich 2015, 31; see also Sherwin-White 1978, 283–285; Buraselis 2000, 66–110; Samama 2003, nos. 142–147). In Lycia, Phrygia, and at Nysa in Asia Minor, wealthy doctors paid for the erection of temples and other monuments in honour of Asclepius (Sherwin-White 1978, 553 note 530; Nutton 2005, 281; Wickkiser 2008, 56–57).

Galen, the most renowned physician of Graeco-Roman antiquity after Hippocrates, who lived in the second century CE and became the doctor of Marcus Aurelius, emphasized his personal relationship with Asclepius. Galen was born in Pergamum. He studied and practised the medical art in his motherland, and perhaps held a post in the local cult of Asclepius before travelling throughout the Roman Empire. He claimed that he was an offspring of the divine physician who had healed his abscess, and moved him to practise medicine (Gal. *Libr. Propr.* 2, 19.18–19K). According to his narrative, the god revealed to his father in a dream that Galen would become a doctor (Gal. *Meth. Med.* 10. 609). Asclepius continued to guide Galen during crucial phases of his life (Gal. *Libri. Propr.* 2; see Schlange-Schöningen 2001,

---

34. As Israelowich (2015, 46) points out, 'The association of physicians with Asclepius and Hygieia was part of the Roman inheritance from the Greek world'.
35. The office of *zakoros* usually was held by people who were assigned as guardians of the temple and were also responsible for the sacred fire and for keeping the place clean; see, for example, Dillon 2002, 90.
36. For a catalogue of the C. Stertinius Xenophon's offerings to Asclepius and other 'paternal gods', see Buraselis 2000, 155–159).

233-235; Nutton 2005, 216-229; Wickkiser 2008, 57; Cilliers and Retief 2013, 87; Mattern 2013, 25-27; Israelowich 2015, 56).[37]

In the same period, Aelius Aristides, a famous orator from Smyrna who suffered from chronic illnesses, used to resort to Asclepius and other gods' aid, as well as consulting human doctors in his quest for health.[38] He obviously believed that Asclepius' treatments and medicine could operate together, healing human illnesses and diseases (Aristid. Or. XLVIII, 31-35, XLVII, 57; see further Behr 1968, 44; Lloyd 1979, 41; Temkin 1991, 184-187; Nutton 2005, 276-279; Wickkiser 2008, 57; Downie 2013a, 89-90; Cilliers and Retief 2013, 87, 88; Mattern 2013, 27-28; Israelowich 2015, 60, 63-67; Russell, Trapp and Nesselrath 2016).[39]

The relationship between Asclepian healing and medical therapy was also promoted by the Asclepius cult.[40] As we have seen, stereotypical visual imagery presented Asclepius as a doctor. The myths underlined Asclepius' medical expertise. In the healing inscriptions, Asclepius appeared to act as a doctor applying certain medical means in order to treat his patients (Wickkiser 2008, 54).

This mutual interest to forge an affinity probably had further benefits for both doctors and the Asclepius sanctuaries. On the one hand, the physicians' dedications probably contributed to the sanctuaries' prosperity, and even the architectural expansion of some *asclepieia* (Samama 2003, 64-66; Wickkiser 2008, 57). On the other hand, as Wickkiser (2008, 57) aptly points out, the display of those dedications in the sanctuaries contributed to the salience and fame of the doctors who honoured their divine colleague. Thus, Asclepius and human doctors appeared to be on the same side, sharing common interests, goals and practices. Furthermore, the

---

37. On the life of Galen, see further Temkin 1973, 10-63; Singer 1997, vii-xliii; Schlange-Schöningen 2001, on the relationship between Galen and Asclepius, esp. 233-235; Mattern 2013; on Galen as a 'neuroscientist and neurophilosopher', see Baloyannis 2016.

38. For Aelius Aristides' biographical information, see, for example, Phillips 1952, 23-25; Behr 1968, 1-25; Miller 1998, 184, 186-187; Horstmanshoff 2004b, 285-286; Holmes 2008, 86; Israelowich 2012, 11-15; Stephens 2012, 76-78).

39. Compare, for instance, an inscription possibly from the *asclepieion* in Cibyra (in southern Phrygia) dated in the second or first century BCE: 'Gratitude to the god for it is cured – and to Tuche of the city and to Dionysius, son of Dionysus the physician who cured me' (Samama 2003, no. 274, cited by Israelowich 2015, 48).

40. Of course, there were cases in which Asclepius appeared to reject the treatments and remedies suggested by human doctors; see, for example, Aristid. Or. XLVII 61-64, 67-68, cf. 54-7, XLIX 79; cf. Lloyd 1979, 46. And there were also doctors who rejected the temple medicine and incubation and were not open to cooperation; see Harris 2009, 185.

Asclepius cult and Hippocratic medicine could be considered to be products of the same development, which differentiated medical orthodoxy from magical practices (Nutton 2005, 112-114; see also Horstmanshoff 2004a, 289-290; Panagiotidou 2016c).

Medical Pluralism, Healing Options and Cultural Expectations in the Graeco-Roman World

As we have seen, Hippocratic medicine and the Asclepius cult constituted alternative but often overlapping healing options that people of the Graeco-Roman world had at their disposal, when they faced health issues (see Lloyd 1979, 40-41). Simultaneously, other healing alternatives developed and coexisted, contributing to the medical pluralism of Graeco-Roman antiquity (see Oberhelman 2013, 1-2, 2014, 47-48).[41] According to Kleinman (1980, 50), healthcare developing in different historical settings comprises 'a local cultural system composed of three overlapping parts: the popular, the professional, and the folk sector'.[42]

In the Graeco-Roman world, along with the doctors that comprised the professional part of healthcare, other kinds of healers claimed their ability to heal the sick for a fee and comprised the folk sector. Root-cutters (ῥιζοτόμοι), drug-sellers (φαρμακοπῶλαι) and the *farmakides* witches (φαρμακίδες) acquired practical knowledge of the medicinal properties of herbs and plants that they sold for curing certain illnesses and diseases (Lloyd 1979, 38-39, 1983, 119-135; Scarborough 1991, esp. 139, 144, 150-152; Gordon 1995, 363; McNamara 2003-2004, 5, 11; Oberhelman 2013, 8; Steger 2018, 20-28). Other healers claimed their ability to heal through the power of their hands or their words, and used purifications and incantations as healing methods. These purifiers (καθάρται), midwives (μαῖαι) and sorcerers (γόαι) as well as priests, diviners and magicians travelled from city to city, much as doctors used to do, offering their services to suffering persons (see, for example, Lloyd 1979, 38, 1983, 119-135; Burkert 1992, 41-43; Dickie 2001, 2010, 88-92, 104-06, 111-112; McNamara 2003-2004,

---

41. Compare the notion of market which has been metaphorically employed to the healthcare system of the Roman Empire by Steger 2018, 9-16.
42. For an application of Kleinman's theory to the Asclepius cult, see Panagiotidou 2016c. On the interaction and intersection between the different kinds of healthcare during the Graeco-Roman era, see also Downie 2013a, 89.

2, 5, 11; Oberhelman 2013, 7-8). They interpreted human diseases as sent by the gods, and promised cure by appealing to divine interventions (McNamara 2003-2004, 11).

The Hippocratic doctors strived to prove their superiority over the folk healers. The works collected in the *Corpus Hippocraticum* – the most renowned medical collection of Greek antiquity – express the doctors' attitudes and opinions towards their profession as a particular kind of art (*techne*) that should be studied, taught and practised (Lloyd 1979, 39-40; Nutton 2005, 62-63; Wickkiser 2008, 22-23; Israelowich 2015, 52). In addition, they reflect a general interest in medicine[43] and the discussions about the role of doctors in the treatment of patients that would have taken place in the popular domain from the fifth century BCE onwards (Demand 1994, 34-36; Nutton 2005, 62; Wickkiser 2008, 23).[44]

The author of *de Morbo Sacro* (the *Sacred Disease*)[45] rigorously attacks those healers that itinerated from city to city, and although they used to observe the symptoms of illnesses and to prescribe certain diets and baths, they attributed the diseases to the gods instead of the human body (Lloyd 1979, 40; Nutton 2005, 65). Particularly the author refers to epilepsy and its characterization as the *sacred disease*, and argues that the brain and not the gods are responsible for this impairment (see, for example, Lloyd 1979, 47-48; van der Eijk 2005, 45; Wickkiser 2008, 24; Israelowich 2015, 52).[46] He wrote:

---

43. This interest is implied by the audience to which these treatises were addressed and ranged from prospective students and individuals with certain interests to actual practitioners and intellects already studying the medical art (Nutton 2005, 62; Wickkiser 2008, 23; Downie 2013a, 93-94).
44. The defence of medicine by the authors of *de Arte* (*on Medical Art*) (1, VI, 2) and *de Vetere Medicina* (*on Ancient Medicine*) (I, 1-2) against the sceptics, implies that the validity of the medical art and the authority of doctors were not yet universally accepted (see Nutton 2005, 63; Harris 2009, 185). Later, during the Graeco-Roman period, doctors comprised a distinctive professional class of high esteem; on the authoritative figures of professional physicians in the Roman society, see Israelowich 2014, 454-455, 2015, 15-18.
45. The polemical attitude of the author towards magicians and other kinds of itinerant healers is evident throughout his work: e.g. 1.2, 1.11-19, 1.25-6, 1.45-6, 2.6-7, 11.5, 12.2, 13.13, 17.1-10, 18.1-2; see van der Eijk 2005, 45-46. On discussions of *de Morbo Sacro* and the author's religious beliefs, see further Roselli 1996; Hankinson 1998a; Wöhlers 1999; Laskaris 2002; Lloyd 2003, 43-50; van der Eijk 2005, 60-70.
46. On the history of epilepsy, see Temkin 1971, esp. 6-10 on the perception of epilepsy as a sacred disease.

> It seems to me that it was people like today's magicians, purifiers, charlatans, and quacks who first made this disease a 'holy' one. It's just those sorts of people who claim to be especially holy and to know a lot. At a loss and having nothing to offer in the way of help, they alleged that the divine was the true cause of this disease and, so as not to appear completely ignorant, called it sacred ... But the cause of this illness is the brain, just as with the other major illnesses; ... they profess to be possessed of superior knowledge, and deceive mankind by enjoining lustrations and purifications upon them, while their discourse turns upon the divinity and the godhead. And yet it would appear to me that their discourse savors not of piety, as they suppose, but rather of impiety, and as if there were no gods, and that what they hold to be holy and divine, were impious and unholy ... For, if they profess to know how to bring down the moon, darken the sun, induce storms and fine weather, and rains and droughts, and make the sea and land unproductive, and so forth, whether they arrogate this power as being derived from mysteries or any other knowledge or consideration, they appear to me to practice impiety, and either to fancy that there are no gods, or, if there are, that they have no ability to ward off any of the greatest evils. How, then, are they not enemies to the gods?
>
> (Hippoc. *Morb. Sacr.* 1.28–30 and 1.39ff., trans. Jones 1923)

According to the author, those itinerant healers obviously believed that the gods were the reason behind human pollution, and it was also the gods who were called upon to resolve the reasons for the pollution (Hippoc. *Morb. Sacr.* 1, 41–43; see further Nutton 2005, 65; van der Eijk 2005, 60, 65–67; Wickkiser 2008, 30–32). However, the belief in the divine origins of diseases and other disabilities is innately blasphemous. And the people who pretend that they are able to manipulate the gods in order to heal their clients are impious as well (Hippoc. *Morb. Sacr.* esp. 1.28–30 and 1.39ff; van der Eijk 2005, 48, 60).

The gods called upon by the Hippocratic doctors were still inherently holy and preserved the cosmic order. Part of this order is the human microcosm. The causes of human illnesses and diseases are natural and can be found in the external conditions which affect people, like weather, water, etc. However, since nature is part of the universal divine order, the origins of the illnesses and disease could be considered as divine as well:[47]

---

47. The divinity of the disease does not entail a novel theology according to which 'nature is the divine'. The diseases can be divine in virtue of their nature (*physes*) or their external causes (*prophaseis*). Van der Eijk (2005) argues that the Hippocratics perceived the divinity of the diseases on account of their *physes*. Jouanna (2003, 130–131), on the other hand,

'And the disease called the Sacred arises from causes as others, namely, those things which enter and exit the body, such as cold, the sun, and the winds, which are changing and are never at rest. And these things are divine' (Hippoc. *Morb. Sacr.* 18, trans. Jones 1923).

This perception of illness and disease, shared by many authors of the *Corpus Hippocraticum*, constituted an obvious shift from previous beliefs which perceived the gods as the origins of human trials, and further changed the ways in which the restoration of health was sought by doctors. Instead of attempting to appease the deities, health could be restored through adjustments of diet, environmental conditions, and other external elements which affect humans (Hippoc. *Morb. Sacr.* 18.3; see van der Eijk 2005, 60; Wickkiser 2008, 31; Kleisiaris, Sfakianakis and Papathanasiou 2014; Israelowich 2015, 52-53). In their attempt to challenge the sceptics who denied the utility of medicine based on the argument that recovery from illnesses is possible without physicians' involvement, while death can happen despite the medical interventions, the Hippocratic authors contrasted medicine to nature and chance by pointing out the progress and discoveries made by the doctors through empirical observations and thorough inquiry. Instead of leaving people's health to chance, doctors looked for the causes of the diseases and tried to understand the links between the things in the external world and the human body (Hippoc. *Art.* 1; *VM* I, 1-2; Kleisiaris, Sfakianakis and Papathanasiou 2014). Once they recognized these causes and links, they were able to apply the appropriate treatments or remedies in order to ensure recovery, when this was feasible (Nutton 2005, 63; see *Hippoc. Flat.* 1, 4; Jouanna 1999, sect. ii, 3; cf. Lloyd 1979, 49-58, 1987, 114-24; Demand 1994, 34-6; Hankinson 1998b, 51-69).

Despite their hostile attitudes towards the religious and magical healers, the authors of the *Corpus Hippocraticum* did not totally reject divine interventions in certain circumstances.[48] For instance, the author of the *de Morbo Sacro* admits that a visit to a god's sanctuary might help eliminate the pollution which a person had caused to him or herself (see van der Eijk

---

suggests that there is no discrepancy between the perception of the divinity of the disease on account of its *physes* or its *prophaseis*; see further Nutton 2005, 65; van der Eijk 2005, 45-46, 60; Wickkiser 2008, 30-32; Israelowich 2015, 52.

48. All the Hippocratic treatises do not share the same beliefs and attitudes towards gods and divine treatments. Possibly, there might also have been doctors who rejected the usefulness of praying to the gods, etc. However, there is no preserved evidence that might confirm the latters' attitudes. Therefore, their beliefs might not have been predominant; see Lloyd 1979, 41-42, 48; Wickkiser 2008, 33.

2005, 60-70; Wickkiser 2008, 31-32; Oberhelman 2014, 48). In this passage, he suggests prayers and sacrifices as the appropriate way to approach the god instead of the practices applied by his contemporaries and the purifiers:

> who ought to do the very reverse, namely, sacrifice and pray, and, bringing gifts to the temples, supplicate the gods. But now they do none of these things, but purify; and some of the purifications they conceal in the earth, and some they throw into the sea, and some they carry to the mountains where no one can touch or tread upon them. But these they ought to take to the temples and present to the god, if a god be the cause of the disease.
> (Hippoc. *Morb. Sacr.* 1, 36-39, trans. C. D. Adams)

Other Hippocratics also appear to be pious, leaving some room for divine healing. According to the author of the Book IV of *Regimen*[49] when an infliction by an illness or a disease is revealed in dreams, prayer of course is suitable but not enough to restore a person to health (Lloyd 1979, 42; Wickkiser 2008, 33). A person has also to take action and change his or her way of living, and dieting along with the appeal to divine aid: 'Prayer indeed is good, but while calling on the gods a man should himself lend a hand' (*Regim.* IV 87, trans. Jones 1923).

This admission of divine help as a supplement to medical practices was accompanied by the acceptance that medicine could not cure all diseases and illnesses. The author of the *Prognostic I* admits doctors' impotence to restore all patients to health: 'For it is impossible to make all the sick well' (Hippoc. *Progn.* I,[50] trans. Adams 1868).

Although the Hippocratic doctors achieved great advances in the medical art, they simultaneously accepted that in cases of incurable diseases, which were inevitably fatal or chronic, or when the progress of a disease had passed its curable point, the medical procedures and treatments were no longer sufficient to ensure recovery.[51] Awareness of these limits

---

49. On the division of *Regimen* in four books, see Jouanna 1999, 408-409.
50. On the date of this treatise, see Jouanna 1999, App. 348.
51. The author of *Prorrheticus* 2 defines in which cases gout cannot be cured by human art: 'As for patients with gout, those who are old, or who have concretions about the joints, or who live a life without exertions and are constipated, are all incurable by the human art, as far as I know' (trans. Potter 1995); the author of *de Morbo Sacro* (2, 2) asserts the limits of medicine arguing that epilepsy can be cured as any other disease, unless it has progressed to such a degree that the remedies cannot fight it any more: 'But this disease seems to me to be no more divine than others; but it has its nature such as other diseases have, and a

entailed the recognition that medicine cannot treat all the possible illnesses and diseases and could not be applied to the conditions which were beyond its power (Hippoc. *Art.* 14). The author of *de Arte* stresses the necessity to abide by the limits of medicine as one of the human arts:[52]

> For if a person expects art to have power in matters where art is not, or expects nature to have power in matters where it is not present, then he is ignorant of an ignorance more in tune with madness than with lack of learning. For those things that we can master using the instruments of art and nature, we can be craftsmen. Of other things, we cannot.
> (Hippoc. *Art.* 8.3, trans. Mann 2012)

In any case, doctors who were professionals with specific social and economic interests, would not risk their good name by taking on patients with incurable diseases (Demand 1994, 45; Jouanna 1999, 107-111; Wickkiser 2008, 25; see further Cohn-Haft 1956, 17-18; Lloyd 1979, 48-49; Von Staden 1990; Prioreschi 1992; Steger 2018, 9-13).[53] The stance of doctors towards individual health conditions would have been evaluated in the popular domain in which certain ideas, beliefs and expectations of the available healing alternatives developed. According to Kleinman (1980, 50), the popular sector comprises the greatest part of any healthcare system that consists of people's family and other social networks in which empirical knowledge about illnesses and diseases, as well as about possible cures and healing options is accumulated and circulates among individuals.[54]

---

cause whence it originates, and its nature and cause are divine only just as much as all others are, and it is curable no less than the others, unless when, the from of time, it is confirmed, and has became stronger than the remedies applied' (trans. Adams 1868; cf. Cilliers and Retief 2013, 74).

52. Various dispositions towards incurable diseases can be traced among the authors of the *Corpus Hippocraticum*. Some of them made a distinction between the treatments which aimed at alleviating suffering, and those which focused on full recovery (Lloyd 1979, 48-49; Patton 2004, 198-199; Wickkiser 2008, 25-26). On the distinction between the different aims of treatment, see Von Staden 1990; Prioreschi 1992, 346; Amundsen 1996, 30-49.

53. Galen claims that the ability of physicians to cure patients suffering from serious diseases is a proof of their medical competence, while a doctor's preference to treat patients with minor ailments entails the lack of skills (*Opt. Med. Cognos.* 14.3). In the same vein, failing to treat patients with incurable diseases would have implied a doctor's unskillfulness and medical incompetence; cf. Petridou 2014, 2018, 2016.

54. Along with professional doctors and folk healers, ordinary people would have shared popular ideas about the medicinal properties and uses of various herbs, plants and natural remedies (see, for example, Plin, *HN* XII-XXVII; cf. Stannard 1982; Scarborough 1991,

Therefore, it was in the popular domain to which people of Graeco-Roman antiquity would have resorted in order to make a choice between professional doctors and folk healers. The patients would have in turn provided feedback for the received treatments formulating the popular ideas and cultural expectations about the various kinds of health providers and the employed healing methods (Kleinman 1980, 50-53; Oberhelman 2013, 3-4; Panagiotidou 2016c; cf. Edelstein and Edelstein 1998, II, 165; Israelowich 2015, 51-52; Epictetus, Dissert. IV, 8, 28-29; Ar. Plut. 400-414, 633-747). Thus, successful cures and good training as well as the ability for *prognoses* – for anticipating the progress and outcome of certain diseases – would have been criteria that distinguished good physicians from the unqualified and other kinds of practitioners and would have contributed to the reputation of medical experts (Wickkiser 2008, 26-27; see further Amundsen 1977; Lloyd 1979, 89, 1987, 39-41).

The healing deities and heroes lay between the professional and folk medicine[55] and comprised a kind of religious alternative that owed its popularity to social interaction and communication of people's empirical knowledge and proclaimed personal experiences of divine interventions. Particularly, Asclepius' healing abilities intersected both the professional and folk sectors by combining official medical training and knowledge with superhuman or even supernatural healing powers (see Panagiotidou 2016c). In mythical sagas, he was classified in the ontological category of persons, and there was nothing counterintuitive in his figure. Simultaneously, his medical training and competence classified him in the cultural category of doctors. In the mythical context, the resurrection of the dead constituted a double violation of both intuitive expectations pertaining to human abilities to win over death and cultural expectations of what the art of medicine can achieve. After his deification, Asclepius abided by the limits of the medical art, as good physicians owed to do. But again, he appeared to surpass his mortal disciples by admitting to heal even the most difficult conditions that doctors had failed or denied to cure and by employing the most advanced healing methods in unexpected ways.

143-144) as well as about particular illnesses and diseases that could be cured by ordinary means. When these means were not enough to restore health, people could search for available alternatives in their environments (Kleinman 1980, 50-53; Panagiotidou 2016c).

55. It's perhaps necessary to emphasize once again that the distinctions between the different sectors of the healthcare system are not rigorous, and the lines between professional medicine, folk healing and popular medical practices intersected and overlapped with one another; see Oberhelman 2014, 47-48.

These violations of cultural expectations of medical practices would have contributed to the diffusion of the beliefs in Asclepius' healing powers and to the popularity of his cult. According to Porubanova-Norquist and her colleagues (2013, 2014), concepts that violate cultural expectations tend to grab people's attention and to be kept in memory and recalled having similar effects with the violations of intuitive expectations.

By minimally violating both intuitive and cultural expectations shared by people of the Graeco-Roman world, the ideas and beliefs in Asclepius' healing powers were culturally transmitted and gradually contributed to the reputation of the supreme divine physician who superseded many minor healing deities and heroes (see, for example, Edelstein and Edelstein 1998, v. II, 89, 119; Nutton 2005, 106–108). He signified not only the divine superhuman healing power, but also the efficacy of medical practices as opposed to religious and magical healing methods. Human doctors, from their own perspective, found in their patron god the divine authentication of their art. For the doctors to repudiate Asclepius would mean that they renounced their own art, means and practices. Thus, the Asclepius cult and professional medicine followed a more or less parallel development, and the interactions and intersections between them continued until the end of the Roman period (Nutton 2005, 113–114; Wickkiser 2008, 57; Cilliers and Retief 2013, 74; Downie 2013a, 89; Israelowich 2015, 51–52).

Symbolic Communication, Dreaming and the Ritual of Incubation

I have suggested that minimally counterintuitive features as well as concepts that mildly violated common cultural expectations would have attracted people's attention to Asclepius and would have increased the salience of the anthropomosphisized physician in the religious life and healthcare system of Graeco-Roman antiquity. What however would have retained people's long-term interest in the divine healer was his special concern in the human well-being, his willingness to help those who suffered from any kind of health problems and his intention to communicate with his supplicants (see Panagiotidou 2016b).

Along with the attribution of other human-like characteristics to perceptible entities, the detection of intentionality in the experienced events and actions constitutes a crucial element of anthropomorphism. Even in the absence of any evident human-like agent, the detection of intentional agency hidden in covered messages, scattered signs or seemingly random events, makes the world less accidental, uncertain and inexplicable and more meaningful, structured and predictable.[56] As Guthrie (1992, 186) points out, religions are grounded on the organization and systematization of an anthropomorphic perception of the world, the design, existence, structure and order of which is attributed to human-like superhuman or supernatural agents who wish to and continually symbolically interact and communicate with humans (Guthrie 1992, 189; cf. Boyer 1996, 89).

Boyer (1996, 90) also endorses the idea that detection of intentionality comprises an essential element of an anthropomorphic perception and interpretation of the world that receives more systematic form in various religious traditions. In addition, Boyer (1996, 89) suggests that the transfer of the psychological trait of intentionality from the ontological category of persons to entities classified in other ontological categories is enough to entail an anthropomorphic perception of these entities. Furthermore, the attribution of any other human-like biological or physical quality to non-human agents inevitably entails the ascription of intentionality, which is the major prerequisite and criterion of religious anthropomorphism (cf. Guthrie 1992, 189; Beerden 2013, 24).

From this perspective, what would have contributed to the ancient Greek gods and goddesses' particular salience in people's lives, was their constant willingness to interact and communicate with humans. The divine messages and interventions in human affairs were considered to be omnipresent in both natural phenomena and everyday individual experiences and social events. Gods, however, usually did not communicate with humans directly, but in covered, symbolic ways that might be untraceable by ordinary people, thus demanding more elaborate means of interpretation. Therefore, divination developed into a craft which promised that it could uncover the meanings and divine messages in the surrounding world and unfolding events and to predict the future.[57]

In particular, practices of natural divination[58] were mainly employed in the ancient Greek oracles, which were popular for claiming that they

---

56. Numerous studies, for instance, explore the human tendency to attribute intentionality to animals' behaviours; see, for example, Heyes and Dickinson 1990; Marler and Ristau 1990; Kennedy 1992, 89; Bekoff, Allen and Burghardt 2002.
57. On ancient Greek divination, see, for example, Bonnechere 2007; Flower 2008; Johnston 2008; Beerden 2013; Panagiotidou 2018; Xygalatas in press.
58. On the distinction between natural and artificial divination, see Cicero, *De Divinatione*, l.12; cf. further Linderski 1982; Denyer 1985; Beard 1986; Schofield 1986; Krostenko 2000; Flower 2008, 85; Johnston 2008, 9–17.

could reveal the future and the divine will through direct communication with the deities. In the face of a significant turning point or in confronting a dilemma crucial for their lives, people could make the decision to consult one of the great oracles of Greek antiquity[59] in order to ask for the gods' opinions of their private matters. Similarly, cities could send delegations to the oracles for significant public affairs (see, for example, Parker 1985; Bremmer 1994, 32–33). There, the priests or priestess, usually reaching some altered states of consciousness resembling ecstasy, claimed that they directly communicated with the gods, who revealed to them their will, predictions and the future consequences of people's actions. However, consulting the oracles was a costly decision in terms of both time and money and was not feasible for every event that people desired to better understand and interpret (Ustinova 2013, 32–34; Xygalatas in press).

For such everyday matters and urgent demands, various practices of artificial divination developed that did not depend on direct communication with the deities, but were intended to trace omens and interpret the divine signs scattered in the physical and social surroundings. Artificial divination was based on the premise that there is a sympathetic relationship between the human and the divine realms which can be revealed, making the perceivable world more conceivable and manageable. Various sorts of seers were trained to detect this sympathetic relationship to every component and aspect of the physical world that might operate as a covert bearer of symbolic communication, and to perform different kinds of technical operations revealing the god's messages (Martin 2004, 159–160; cf. Flower 2008; Johnston 2008, 109–143). Thus, it was believed that omens and divine messages were hidden almost everywhere: in the water, the clouds and the air, in the flight of the birds, in animals' behaviours and the entrails of sacrificial victims, that could be traced by those who exerted respectively the crafts of hydromancy, nephomancy and

---

59. Among the most popular ancient Greek Oracles were those of Apollo in Delphi, in Delos, and in Didyma (Miletos), as well as the Oracles of Zeus in Olympia (Peloponnese) and Dodona (Epeirus). These Oracles were of high esteem, and their prophecies were considered to be more valid than those given to less prestigious sanctuaries. For that reason, they attracted so many visitors who often had to wait their turn for long in order to consult the priests or priestesses (Xygalatas in press; see also Bonnechere 2007, 147–150; Flower 2008, 2; Johnston 2008, 33–108; Stoneman 2011; on the attempts to attract more visitors and the competition between the Oracles see Eidinow 2014).

aeromancy, ornithomancy, theriomancy and hieroscopy.[60] Divine signs could also be found even in accidental events – such as words randomly uttered (cledonism or cledomancy) – or in natural phenomena – such as earthquakes, eclipses, lightning and thunderbolts, plagues and diseases – that occasionally struck people. Since every natural phenomenon, physical substance, chance event or human action was thought to carry meaning and possible exceptional significance for both private citizens and social communities, it was not possible for the latter to continually consult professional seers or the oracles in order to be informed about the divine will and their own future. Thus, people themselves used various ordinary practices and techniques in order to make sense of things happening to them and to find deeper meanings, reasons and significance in seemingly random events and experiences (see Beerden 2013, 23, 55–61).

Among all those sorts of conditions and chance events which were believed to carry divine signs and messages, there was a universal type of private experience, shared by all humans, covered by a veil of mystery that provided the ground for divination. It was in the realm of dreams which were considered to be a gate (or gates)[61] through which the gods communicated with humans in a transient state of consciousness. But not all dreams were considered to be prophetic or oracular, demanding interpretation. There were also non-prophetic dreams that were simply the products of the human mind that processes recent experiences, mental states and bodily activities during sleep.[62] Oneiromancy was the technique

---

60. Omens could be found in every natural substance, physical entity or practice employed by humans, an idea that entails that everything in the world is full of meaning. Thus, numerous methods of divination developed including botanomancy, daphnomancy, molybdomancy, tephromancy, ceromancy, cephalonomancy, sideromancy, causinomancy, osteomancy, crystallomancy, rhabdomancy, catoptromancy, dactylomancy, axinomancy, aleuromancy, alectromancy, lithomancy, onychomancy and so on. Aeschylus in his *Prometheus Desmotes* (*Prometheus Bound*) briefly summarizes the major sorts of the divinatory craft; see, for example, Flower 2008, 89–90; Beerden 2013, 22–23; for an account of the ancient and modern Greek practices of divination, see Xygalatas in press.

61. Ancient Greeks distinguished between significant dreams, which could come true, and insignificant ones, which could prove to be deceptive. In the *Odyssey* (xix, 560–567), Homer draws a distinction between true dreams which reach consciousness through the gate of horn, and others that deceive people passing through the gate of ivory.

62. As we shall see in the fifth chapter, the Hippocratic author of the *Regimen* IV was the first to draw a distinction between prophetic dreams sent by the gods and dreams deriving from the body and the mind which can be used as diagnostic tools by physicians. Plato (*Ap.* 33c) also separated those dreams which were sent by the gods who wished to communicate

used to interpret those dreams that were believed to have been sent by the gods. There were experts who could distinguish between prophetic and non-prophetic dreams and who could be consulted by the dreamers about the meanings and significance of their dreams.[63]

A specific kind of dreams, considered to be particularly important and used as a means of both natural and artificial divination, were the healing dreams that were solicited during the ritual of incubation practised in the sanctuaries of healing deities and especially of Asclepius (see Ferguson 2003, 221-222; Israelowich 2015, 5, 53-54; Renberg 2017, 3, 27-28, 115-116). The incubants of Asclepius expected to have direct communication from the god during sleep. Some of them reported that they had received the desired dream during which the god directly healed them or prescribed the appropriate remedy to them. Others claimed that they had received oracular dreams which needed decoding and interpretation by the experts – usually the priests of the god. In any case, the healing dreams, or visions, were the main gate through which the divine healer was believed to appear and communicate with his supplicants, perform

---

with humans from those dreams which derived from the bodily milieu and displayed internal disturbances and problems (Pl. *Ti.* 45e). Those dreams which were considered to be both true and god-sent were the most significant and demanded interpretation. Aristotle (*Insomn.* 462b12-17) and Epicurus (*Sent. Vat.* 24) disputed the divine origins of dreams and their prophetic qualities and looked for the natural causes and impacts of dreaming. In the last chapter, I shall examine how the cognitive processes that underlie dreaming experiences would have generated the divine dreams and visions in the *asclepieia*.

63. Artemidorus' *Oneirocritica* is the only ancient Greek study about dreams which still exists in its entirety. Artemidorus makes the distinction between *oneiros* (ὄνειρος) and *enhypnion* (ἐνύπνιον) and approaches the ordinary dreams, excluding the oracular dreams from his study, written in the second century CE; see, for example, Lloyd 1979, 43; Holowchak 2002, 94-96; Du Bouchet and Chandezon 2012; Harris-McCoy 2012. Ordinary people possibly used these words, *oneiros* and *enhypnion*, as synonyms (see Harrisson 2013, 64 referring to Leuci 1993, 214). The role of dreams in the therapeutic practices of the Hellenistic era is the main theme of Aelius Aristides' *Orationes* (*Sacred Tales*). He considers dreams to be a means of divine revelation, and mainly focuses on his dreams about his health problems, which received treatment from Asclepius; on Aelius Aristides see, for example, Phillips 1952, 23-25; Behr 1968; Miller 1998, 184, 186-187; Petsalis-Diomidis 2010; Horstmanshoff 2004b, 285-286; Harris and Holmes 2008; Israelowich 2012; Stephens 2012. On the prophetic and somatic dreams, see Behr 1968, 174; Lloyd 1979, 43; Miller 1998, 93, 96, 113; Martin 2004, 174; Harris 2009; Harrisson 2013; Israelowich 2015, 53-54, 68.

his treatments or express his will and the future outcomes of patients' conditions.[64]

Healing dreams and visions were the most common means through which Asclepius appeared to his supplicants and provided cures. As I suggest in the following chapters, however, along with the anthropomorphized appearances of Asclepius in his supplicants' sleep, often reported in the inscriptions from the *asclepieia*, the patients who visited the temples were predisposed to recognize his incarnation in other entities – like in his sacred animals, the snakes and the dogs – or even to trace his invisible presence in seemingly accidental events. In any case, what mainly attracted visitors to the *asclepieia* and contributed to the popularity of the sanctuaries, was the patients' belief that Asclepius was eager and strongly desired to communicate and heal his supplicants, revealing his remedies and prescriptions that would lead them to recovery and salvation.

---

64. Prophetic messages and information deriving from the body were sought in the healing dreams evoked during incubation, since they were considered to be revelations made by the god regarding his supplicants' health issues (see Cilliers and Retief 2013, 69; Renberg 2017, 28).

Chapter 3

The Spread of the Asclepius Cult

Deciding to Visit an *Asclepieion*

Although the early development of the Asclepius cult cannot be fully traced, the archaeological and historical evidence indicates that the cult developed into an organized religious institution in the sixth century BCE and enjoyed increased popularity from the Classical period onwards. Particularly during the Graeco-Roman era, the vast geographical area of the Hellenistic *oecumene*, within which people could move and travel, and later the establishment of the *pax Romana*, formed favourable conditions for the flourish of the great *asclepieia*, where it was believed that Asclepius usually resided (Israelowich 2015, 47, 50).

Within the extended borders of Graeco-Roman world, along with travellers, their ideas, beliefs, and precepts followed, and these developed and passed on through multiple interactions between people and individuals and their external natural, social, representational, and symbolic surroundings. In these cultural contexts, Asclepius was perceived as the benevolent deity who was close to humans, and his healing services were available to everyone who visited his temples, comprising a significant healing option among other healing alternatives.

In this chapter, I outline the geographical expansion of the Asclepius cult and focus on those features shared by the great *asclepieia* that made these sanctuaries attractive healing places for people suffering from health problems. I further examine those motives and conditions that could move persons afflicted by an illness to resort to Asclepius temples and ask for his aid. I do not claim that the scenarios presented in this chapter represent actual cases of patients who behaved in a predetermined way. What I mostly intend is to outline possible routes that people's minds could move along, ending up visiting an Asclepius temple. In this light, visiting an *asclepieion* was one among other healing options provided by the medical pluralism of the Graeco-Roman world, which patients could freely choose, without the obligation of following a fixed hierarchy (e.g. to consult first a doctor and afterwards Asclepius). Moreover, the healing inscriptions noted here are not taken at face value, but are mainly approached as rhetorical means used by cult authorities in order to predict and manipulate supplicants' reactions. Thus, I suggest that personal feelings of distress and despair could cause patients who looked for recovery to turn to the divine physician. On the other hand, I explore those social interactions that could have mediated the increase of Asclepius' popularity, taking into account neurocognitive theories of observation of others and of social learning. In this framework, I suggest that, as more patients flocked to the healing sanctuaries, the popularity of these places increased and the reputation of the divine healer spread throughout the Graeco-Roman world.

Asclepius Cult: Appearance and Geographical Expansion

There is only scarce evidence in literary sources about the existence of an Asclepius cult before the sixth century BCE. This evidence indicates that Asclepius was possibly worshipped as a hero or semi-deity in the city of Trikka in Thessaly. In the *Iliad*, Homer mentioned Trikka as the motherland of Asclepius (Hom. *Il.* II, 695). Hesiod (fr. 122 = T. 21) and the author of the *Homeric Hymns* (16, 1–3 = T. 31) also pointed out the connection of Asclepius with Thessaly and the city of Trikka. Later, in the third century BCE, the mime-writer Herondas (*Mim.* IV, 1–95= T. 482) argued that Asclepius arrived in Kos travelling from Trikka. In the second century CE, the geographer Strabo (*Geog.* VIII, 4, 4, IX, 5, 17 = T. 714, 715, 767) also refers to Trikka as the place where the earliest and most popular sanctuary of Asclepius was located (see Dillon 1994, 242; Edelstein and Edelstein 1998, v. II, 71; Nutton 2005, 104–105; Wickkiser 2008, 35–36; Renberg 2017, 202–203). However, the references in literary works have not been testified by archaeological findings, since archaeologists have not yet found this archaic sanctuary.[1] In any case, even if the Asclepius cult originated from the city of Trikka in the archaic era, his reputation expanded and

---

1. Insufficient evidence is provided by Julius Ziehen (1892, 195–197). Kastriotis (1918, 65–67) discovered a *stoa*, but it is dated in late Hellenistic period.

reached Epidaurus in Peloponnese quite early, where the most significant of his sanctuaries was established.

The cult of Asclepius appeared in Epidaurus at the end of the sixth century BCE, when the first *asclepieion* was built near a spring some distance from the pre-existing Apollo Maleatas sanctuary.[2] Asclepius was the master of the sanctuary, and he was worshipped as the ultimate healing deity. However, his connection with Apollo was most obvious in this region, and he was worshipped alongside his father (Martin and Metzger 1992, 105–110; see Renberg 2017, 173–174). By the early fourth century BCE, the Asclepius sanctuary in Epidaurus attracted supplicants from numerous cities. The inscriptions record patients coming from Aigina, Argos, Halieis, Epeirus, Messene, Sparta, Herakleia, Hermione, Kaphyiai, Keos, Chios, Kirrha, Knidos, Lampsakos, Mytilene, Pherai, Thasos, Thebes, Torone and Troezen (see, for example, Dillon 1994, 243, 1997, 73–80; Wickkiser 2008, 41).[3] The popularity of the sanctuary further increased the prosperity of the priesthood. The early sanctuary was extensively restored in order to host even more supplicants (Martin and Metzger 1992, 109–114; Papachatzis 2002, 205; Riethmüller 2005, v. I, 279–324).[4] A magnificent building complex was constructed and decorated with unique works of art. In this manner, the Epidaurian priesthood might have attempted to prove the superiority of the sanctuary over other Asclepius cult centres, most of which were established under its direct influence (Martin and Metzger 1992, 114; see further Burford 1969).

Gradually, the belief that Asclepius was born in Thessaly was forgotten, and Epidaurus was widely accepted as the place of the god's origin in the people's minds (Julian. *C. Galil.* 200 A-B; Marin. *V. Pr.* Cp. 31; Lactant. *St.i Theb.* III). The recognition of Epidaurus as the motherland of Asclepius was validated by an oracle by Pythia in Delphi. The contention between two of the earliest *asclepieia*, those in Messene (sixth century BCE) (Zunino 1997, 139–189; Themelis 2010) and in Arcadia in Peloponnese (fourth century BCE) (Martin and Metzger 1940-1941, 280–286, 1942-1943, 330–334, 1992, 78, 85; cf. Ginouvès 1959), provided the possibility of such affirmation. These regions claimed the god's origins as narrated in different mythical

---

2. Apollo's sanctuary was retained even in the fourth century BCE – a time when the *asclepieion* was at its peak (Martin and Metzger 1992, 105–110).

3. An examination of the geographical diffusion of the Asclepius cult was published in Panagiotidou 2016c.

4. For a more thorough description and analyses of the architecture of the sanctuary, see Roux 1961.

versions of his descent. Messenians, on the one hand, argued that the mother of Asclepius was Arsinoë, the daughter of the Messenian king Leucippus (Paus. *Descr. Graec.* II, 26, 7 = T. 16). Arcadians, on the other hand, claimed that a woman bearing the same name (Arsinoë), but originating from Arcadia, gave birth to Asclepius.[5] The disagreement between the two regions reached the Delphic Oracle when the Arcadian Apollophanes travelled to Delphi in order to ask Pythia for a definitive answer regarding Asclepius' origins. Despite his aspirations, the reply he received rejected both Arcadian and Messenian claims, recognizing Epidaurus as the motherland of the divine healer (Paus. *Descr. Graec.* II, 26, 7 = T. 16; see Edelstein and Edelstein 1998, v. II, 68–69; Nutton 2005, 104–105).

Under the influence of Epidaurus, *asclepieia* were built in Athens[6] and Corinth (see Roebuck 1951; Lang 1977; Martin and Metzger 1992, 75–76; Papachatzis 2002, 80), and became part of the religious life of their citizens in the Classical period (fifth–fourth centuries BCE) (Nutton 2005, 105). In the fourth century BCE, *asclepieia*, based on Epidaurian models, were established in Pergamum in Asia Minor (see, for example, Deubner 1938; Ziegenaus and De Luca 1968; Habicht 1969; Bean 1979, 58–59; McDonagh 1989, 222–225; Hoffmann 1998; Jones 1998; Petsalis-Diomidis 2010, 151–220; Melfi 2016) and Lebena on Crete (see Melfi 2007, 2010) through private initiatives. The *asclepieion* in Pergamum predominated in Asia Minor, and gradually became the second most famous sanctuary of the god, after Epidaurus. According to Philostratus (*V A* 4, 34), the *asclepieion* in Lebena was for Crete what the *asclepieion* in Pergamum was for Asia, and gradually attracted visitors and supplicants not only from areas of the island but also from Libya: 'And this is a shrine of Asclepius, and just as the whole of Asia flocks to Pergamon, so the whole of Crete flocked to this shrine; and many Libyans also cross the sea to visit it, for it faces towards the Libyan

---

5. The mythical saga developed by Arcadians is little known (see Paus. *Descr. Graec.* VIII, 25, 11= T. 17; Edelstein and Edelstein 1998, v. II, 68–69; cf. Polyb. *Hist.* IV, 33.
6. Different explanations have been formulated for the initial arrival of Asclepius to Athens. Herzog (1931, 38) and Edelstein and Edelstein (1998, v. II, 120) attribute the introduction of his cult to a successful private healing. Martin and Metzger (1992, 94) as well as Aleshire (1989) argue that the Athenians invoked Asclepius from Epidaurus after they had been affected by the plague. In any case, the arrival of Asclepius to Athens was the result of an individual initiative. On the Athenian *asclepieion*, see Girard 1831; Martin and Metzger 1949, 316–350; Travlos 1971, 127–137; Papachatzis 2002, 304; Lefantzis and Jensen 2009; Papaefthymiou 2009; Wickkiser 2009; Petridou 2016, 178–179.

sea close to Phaestus, where the little rock keeps out a might sea' (trans. Conybeare 1912 = T. 792).

The cult of Apollo preceded the arrival of Asclepius on Kos. As mentioned in the previous chapter, Hippocrates was also born on Kos in the fifth century BCE, and the medical school he established in his motherland continued to practise medicine long after his death. A sanctuary on Kos was dedicated to Asclepius in the following century, and this Koan *asclepieion* developed into a popular therapeutic centre during the Graeco-Roman era (Martin and Metzger 1992, 79, 106–107; further Herzog 1928; Kerényi 1959, 50–53; Sherwin-White 1978).

In the Hellenistic period, Asclepius' popularity increased rapidly, and numerous temples were erected in his honour in almost every city of the Hellenistic world. The spread of the Asclepius cult was facilitated by the development of a wide network of newly founded Greek cities throughout the known world – from Asia Minor, Syria and Palestine to the eastern regions beyond the Tigris (Billows 2005, 198; cf. Shipley and Hansen 2006). The practice of establishing new cities was inaugurated by Alexander the Great[7] and was continued by his successors,[8] while these regions later comprised urban centres of the vast Roman Empire.[9] Most of these cities were installed on pre-existing native towns or settlements and included local populations. The main purpose of their establishment was the guarding of the remote areas of Alexander's empire, and later of his successor's kingdoms and the Roman Empire. However, these settlements developed to be Greek cities by imposing an element of a Greek population as well as by adopting the political administration, social organization, cultural and religious institutions of the traditional Greek city-states. These cities

---

7. According to Pausanias (*Descr. Graec.* VIII, 28, 1), Alexander the Great offered his honour to Asclepius: 'The natives also say that Alexander the son of Philip dedicated to Asclepius his breastplate and spear. The breastplate and the head of the spear are still there today' (trans. Jones and Ormerod 1918).
8. The establishment of Alexandria in Egypt in 333/332 BCE by Alexander the Great was followed by founding new cities throughout the conquered regions of the former Persian Empire. The Hellenistic monarchs continued this practice and founded numerous cities naming them after themselves (Seleukeia after Seleukos Nikator, Antiocheia after Antiochos and so on; Billows 2005, 197–199; cf. Cohen 1995)
9. The integration of the Greaco-Roman world, which began with the campaigns of Alexander the Great, wholly occurred in 30 CE with the conquest of Egypt by Octavian Augustus, and the establishment of the Roman Empire (see, for example, Nock 1933, 99–102; Seibert 1979; Chamoux 2003; Gehrke 2003, 110–149; Pachis 2003, 29–42, 64–68, 2004, 11–73; Martin 2004, 85–102).

attracted the surplus population of the Greek mainland – people who looked for opportunities to improve their lives away from their homeland. The greatest of these cities gradually developed into cosmopolitan centres where people from different regions gathered, blended with the natives and lived together (see, for example, Rostovtzeff 1941, II, 623–624, 1045–1048; Green 1990, 363–265; Walbank 1999, 85–87; Chamoux 2003, 165–213, 255–322; Pachis 2003, 44, 51). In addition, numerous visitors and itinerant professionals would pass through these Hellenistic cities. Mercenaries (Griffith 1935; Rostovtzeff 1941, I, 143–8, II, 1033, 1126–1127; Green 1990, 39–40, 45–46, 302–303; Walbank 1999, 82–89, 91, 163–166; Gehrke 2003, 144–145; for further literature see Pachis 2003, 53–54; McKechnie 2014), merchants and traders, priests (Burkert 1983, 111–119; Green 1990, 312; Pachis 2003, 55; McKechnie 2014), magicians (Dickie 2010), and physicians wandered from city to city, offering their services and earning money. Thus, the Hellenistic cities developed into messy melting pots where various cultural influences met and blended with each other.[10] In these cultural contexts, social interactions among people of different origins would have contributed to the spread and sharing of cultural representations that they bore with them from their homelands. Such interactions would have mediated the diffusion of beliefs in Asclepius and his healing powers. The establishment of *asclepieia* in most of the cities of the Graeco-Roman world seems to confirm the wide spread of the cult and of beliefs in Asclepius.

During the fourth and third centuries BCE, around 200 sanctuaries were dedicated to Asclepius on mainland Greece.[11] In the Peloponnese, besides Corinth, Messene, Arcadia and Epidaurus, the Asclepius cult spread to Argos (Paus. *Descr. Graec.* II, 21, 1 = T. 751), Cyllene (Paus. *Descr. Graec.* VI, 21, 4 = T. 780), Helieia (Paus. *Descr. Graec.* VI, 26, 5, V, 7, 1 = T. 779, 781), Gortys (Paus. *Descr. Graec.* VIII, 26, 6, X, 32, 12 = T. 774, 719.) and Sicyon (Paus. *Descr. Graec.* II, 10, 2 = T. 747, 774). *Asclepieia* were also built in Attica (Schol. Ar. *Plut.* 621 = T. 722), Phocis (Paus. *Descr. Graec.* X, 34, 6 = T. 718) and Macedonia (see Lioulias 2010).

---

10. On the 'messines' of culture and major theoretical considerations on this idea see Klostergaard Petersen 2009.
11. Riethmüller (2005, v. II, 9–315) numbers 171 *asclepieia* in main Greece and provides valuable discussions about the sites that have been excavated; cf. Semeria 1986.

Hundreds of Asclepius cult centres were established beyond the Greek mainland.[12] *Asclepieia* were built on many Greek islands, e.g. on Euboea (*IG* XII, 9, 194 = T. 787), Thasos (*IG* XII, 8, 265 = T. 786), Delos (*IG* XI, 2, 161 A, 72–73 = T. 788), Paros (*IG* XII, 5, 119 = T. 789) and Anaphe (*IG* XII, 3, 248 = T. 790). In Asia Minor, besides Pergamum, temples were devoted to Asclepius in Bithynia (Paus. *Descr. Graec.* III, 3, 8 = T. 800), Mysia (Aristid. *Or.* L, 3 = T. 812), Lydia (Paus. *Descr. Graec.* VII, 5, 9, XLVII, 17 = T. 813, 814), Caria (Vitr. *De arch.* VII, *Praef.* 12 = T. 815), Cilicia (Philostr. *V A*, I, 7 = T. 816; Lib. *Orat.* XXX, 39 = T. 817; Euseb. *Vit. Const.* III, 56 = T. 818; Sozom. *Hist. eccl.* II, 5 = T. 819; Zonar. *Epit. Hist.* XIII, 12 C–D = T. 820), Media (Arr. *Alex. Anab.* VII, 14, 5–6 = T. 821) and Scythia (Steph. Byz. *Ethn.* s.v. Ἅγιον = T. 822). In Phoenicia, the Asclepius cult is testified in Berytus (Strabo, *Geog.* XVI, 2, 22 = T. 823; Dam. *Isid.* 302 = T. 826) and Sidon (Strabo, *Geog.* XVI, 2, 22 = T. 823; Phil. Bybl. Fr. 2, 20 = T. 825).

In the early third century BCE, the Romans also evoked Asclepius in order to relieve them from the plague that had broken out in their city.[13] In 293 BCE, the Roman priests consulted the Sibylline Books, which revealed that salvation would come, only if they would invoke Asclepius from Epidaurus. The following year, the Roman senate sent an official delegation to Epidaurus, which brought Asclepius to Rome. In 291 BCE, a sanctuary was devoted to Asclepius on the Tiber Island. The plague subsided soon afterwards, and Romans continued to worship the romanized Aesculapius, visiting his temple in order to be cured from their diseases. The *asclepieion* of Tiber Island – also called *aedes*, *templum* (Val. Max. *Fact. Dict. Memor.* I, 8, 2; Ov. *Nas. Fast.* I.290) and *fanum* (Livy, *Ab Urb. Cond.* XLIII, 4) – became particularly popular among slaves, freedmen and freedwomen who gained their freedom after Asclepius took care of them.[14] From then on, the Aesculapius cult spread in Rome and its environs (Renberg 2006/2007,

---

12. Riethmüller (2005, v. II, 317–360) lists 732 centres of the Asclepius cult beyond the main Greece.
13. Main sources about Asclepius' arrival in Rome: Val. Max. *Fac. Dic. Mem.* I, 8, 2 = T. 848; [Aur. Vict.], *De vir. ill.* 22, 1–3 = T. 849; Ov. *Met.* XV, 622–744 = T. 850; Livy, *Per.* XI = T. 846. On the invocation of Asclepius to Rome and the Roman *asclepieion*, see, for example, Kerényi 1959, 5–15; Roesch 1982; Musial 1990; Dillon 1997, 76; Orlin 1997, 106–108; Nutton 2005, 159–161; Riethmüller 2005, v. I, 233–236, v. II, 431–432, no. 586; Renberg 2006/2007, 88–89, 91–105; Glinister 2007, 21–23; Israelowich 2015, 13; Steger 2018, 17–18; van der Ploeg 2018.
14. According to Suetonius (*Claud.* 25 = T. 858), sick and old slaves were abandoned on the Tiber Island by their masters. Asclepius took care of them and those who recovered, gained their freedom.

90–91, 105–114, 2017, 206–208; Panagiotidou 2016c; cf. van der Ploeg 2018). On the Italian peninsula, sanctuaries were also devoted to Asclepius in Fregellae (see Coarelli 1986; Crawford et al. 1986; Morehouse 2012, 39–44) and Tarentum (Julian. *C. Galil.* 200 B = T. 825). In Sicily (Renberg 2006, 113), *asclepieia* were built in Syracuse (Polyaenus, *Strat.* V, 2, 19 = T. 841) and Acragas (Polyb. *Hist.* I, 18, 2 = T. 839; Cic. *Verr.* IV, 43, 93 = T. 840).[15]

In the Graeco-Roman era, in addition to the Eastern regions of the Roman Empire, the Asclepius cult spread in the Latin provinces (Renberg 2006/2007, 88) and reached as far as the Greek settlements in Cyrene and other places of Roman Africa[16] and the Gaul provinces.[17] Roman soldiers and veterans of the Roman army worshipped Asclepius, and temples were established in his honour in military camps and stations (see Renberg 2006/2007, 115–119; Panagiotidou 2016c; van der Ploeg 2018, 166–214).[18]

Contrary to the early sanctuaries, which were mostly established at some distance from the cities,[19] the local Hellenistic and Roman temples of Asclepius were often included in the wider urban settings. The citizens used to visit them in order to pray for their own good health and their families' well-being,[20] attend the daily rituals and ask for the god's help

---

15. For the spread of the Asclepius cult in the Roman Empire and the different agents of dissemination in the Roman provinces, see van der Ploeg 2018, especially chapter 3 ff.
16. In Roman Africa, inscriptions were found in Calama (*ILAlg.* I 176; *CIL* VIII 5288), Theveste (*ILAlg.* I 3066), Madaurus (*ILAlg.* I 2031), Thubursicu Numidarum (*ILAlg.* I 1220), Lambaesis (*CIL* VIII 2579a, 2589, 2590, 2624; *AE* 1967, 571, 1973, 630, 1989, 870), Carthage (*CIL* VIII 25516; *AE* 1968, 553 a.), Mustis (*AE* 1968, 586, 595, 596, 609, 1973, 641) and Balagrae in Cyrenaica (*SEG* 20 759); see Kleijwegt 1994, 209–210. A *lex sacra* (*ILAfr.* 225) was found at Thuburbo Maius in Africa, which determines specific rules and abstentions that supplicants should follow before the ritual of incubation (cf. *IPerg.* VIII, 161, II, 12–14); see Kleijwegt 1994, 210–211; cf. van der Ploeg 2018, 215–262.
17. Inscriptions and reliefs, found in Gaul, were mainly dedicated by Greeks and members of the Roman administration, a fact which indicates that Asclepius was widely worshipped in these regions where there was a significant Greek population; see Renberg 2006, 126–129.
18. Dedications made by Roman soldiers have been found in regions of Gaul, northern Britania and Moesia; see Gordon and Reynolds 2003, 260.
19. The early Messenian *asclepieion* was exceptionally situated within the city. In that region, Asclepius was considered to be a fellow citizen who was born there, and was honoured by the citizens as a local patron deity. The healing features of Asclepius were not prevalent in this sanctuary, as it is indicated by the fact that there was no building appropriate for the enactment of incubation and the healing of the sick (Nutton 2005, 107; see further Habicht 1985, 37–63; Zunino 1997, 139–189, 281–284).
20. For example, two parents made a dedication to Asclepius asking him to protect their daughter from any harm or illness; see Renberg 2006/2007, 112, 124, 147, cat. no. 16.

to resolve their everyday ordeals, and to meet and associate with other people. Local *asclepieia* were connected with the pleasures and miseries of the people of every city (Edelstein and Edelstein 1998, v. II, 233).[21]

In particular, for sick people, it was more convenient to visit a local temple and ask for Asclepius' aid (Dillon 1994, 240, 1997, 76; Edelstein and Edelstein 1998, 234; cf. Renberg 2006/2007, 108). Local *asclepieia* offered patients the opportunity to avoid the expenses and risks of travelling to Asclepius' remote sanctuaries, and thus enhanced the predominant role of the cult in the devotees' lives (Edelstein and Edelstein 1998, v. II, 234; Panagiotidou 2015). Themistius, who wrote his *Orationes* in the fourth century CE, refers to an Asclepius temple which lay in ruins during his time, and emphasized the significance of the local sanctuaries (Edelstein and Edelstein 1998, v. II, 233–234; Panagiotidou 2016c): 'If we were ill in body and required the help of the god, and he was present here in the temple and the acropolis and was offering himself to the sick, just as even of old he is said to have done, would it be necessary to go to Trikka and sail to Epidaurus on account of their ancient fame, or to move two steps and get rid of our illness?' (Them. *Or.* XXVII, trans. Edelstein and Edelstein 1998 = T. 385).

However, the increase in numbers of local temples did not diminish the popularity of the great *asclepieia* in Epidaurus, Pergamum, Lebena, and on Kos. Asclepius' healing power was perceived as more efficacious in these sanctuaries, which eventually developed into pan-Hellenistic healing centres and continued to attract patients during the Roman period (Dillon 1994, 239–240, 1997, 76; Edelstein and Edelstein 1998, v. II, 234; Ferguson 2003, 222–225; Petsalis-Diomidis 2005, 186).

The Great *Asclepieia*: Where Healing Was Possible

From the fourth century BCE onwards, numerous men, women and children from different social classes suffering from various diseases and disabilities resorted to the great sanctuaries of Asclepius expecting a healing dream or vision from the divine physician. Since the offered treatments were free of charge and the god only asked for low-cost thank-offerings

---

21. For example, a couple in Rome wished to thank Asclepius for his help in their bean trade business and made a dedication of two metal tapers in his honour (see Renberg 2006/2007, 112, 135, 146–147, cat. no. 15).

for successful cures (e.g. Herond. *Mim.* IV, 1-95), there were no social or economic restrictions to the range of patients who could ask for Asclepius' aid. Of course, visiting the remote great *asclepieia* presupposed that the supplicants could afford at least the travel expenses and the cost of accommodation (see Edelstein and Edelstein 1998, II, 173-180). As the ancient testimony indicates, the educated of the era – literary men (Suda, s.v. Θεόπομπος = T. 456; see further Edelstein and Edelstein 1998, v. II, 205-208), poets (e.g. Antiphanes; cf. Athen. *Deipnosoph.* XI, 70, 485b = T. 611; Apul. *Flor.* 18 = T. 608), orators (e.g. Aeschines the Rhetor; cf. *Anth. Pal.* VI, 330; Aristid. *Or.*) and philosophers (e.g. Proclus; cf. Marin, *V. Proc.* Cp. 30 = T. 445; Polemon of Smyrna; cf. Philostr. *V S* I, 25, 4 = T. 433; Hermocrates; cf. Philostr. *V S* II, 25, 5 = T. 434) – were among Asclepius' supplicants and promoted the reputation of his temples in their works (see Israelowich 2015, 111-113; Afonasin 2019). Roman officials, even emperors, visited the great *asclepieia* when they had the opportunity. Among them, the emperor Caracalla visited the *asclepieion* in Pergamum desiring a treatment from Asclepius (Hdn. *Exc.essu D. Marc.*, IV, 8, 3 = T. 437; Dio Cass. Dio *Hist. Rom.* 78.16, 7-8; Hdn *Hist. Emp.* 4.8.3).[22] Hundreds of anatomical votive offerings, dedicated by Asclepius' supplicants, as well as records of divine cures preserved in narrative inscriptions have been found and confirm the popularity of the great *asclepieia*. These offerings and inscriptions were exhibited in various places within the sanctuaries, propagating the divine healing power of Asclepius (Holmes 2008, 101; see further Van Straten 1981, 78-79, 1992, 270-272; LiDonnici 1995, 41).

Archaeological excavations have revealed that the *asclepieia* in Epidaurus (Martin and Metzger 1992, 109-114; Riethmüller 2005, vol. I, 229-240), Pergamum (Martin and Metzger 1992, 98, 100-102; Deubner 1938),[23] Lebena (Melfi 2007, 57-58, 62-63) and on Kos (Herzog 1928; Sherwin-White 1978; Martin and Metzger 1992, 79; Chamoux 2003, 335-338) shared characteristics, that seem to have been essential for the Asclepius cult at these centres (see Cilliers and Retief 2013, 70-74; Renberg 2017, 124-125). For example, all the great *asclepieia* were established at some distance from the cities,[24] in or close to groves, while the existence of natural springs or

---

22. A brief examination of the origins and social status of the Asclepius' supplicants has been published in Panagiotidou 2016c.
23. On the sanctuary before the reconstruction of the second century CE, see Ziegenaus and De Luca 1968; on the epigraphic material from this sanctuary, see Habicht 1969.
24. The Epidaurian sanctuary of Asclepius was built about 10 km inland from the city of Epidaurus (Martin and Metzger 1992, 105-110; Melfi 2010, 329). The first *asclepieion* in

a proximity to the sea was essential.[25] The *asclepieia* were developed within the *temenos* – a piece of land that belonged to the god and was demarcated by the holy precinct or milestones. Altars were dedicated to Asclepius and other deities[26] within the *temenos*. A temple of Asclepius was erected, and this hosted his cult statue.[27] A prolonged *stoa* constituted the *enkoimetērion* (ἐγκοιμητήριον), the hall where the ritual of incubation took place. This *stoa* was the *abaton* of the temple, where only the patients who had followed all the preparatory steps could enter in order to sleep over night, in the hope of experiencing a healing dream from Asclepius.[28] Fountains were built, which supplied the sanctuaries with water for the purification rituals and therapeutic practices. In addition, for the adequate water supply, aqueduct systems were constructed including channels and tubes, which provided a continuous flow of water in the fountains (cf. Panagiotidou 2013, 2021a).[29] Baths were often constructed for personal hygiene, as well as therapeutic purposes (Figure 2).

Plutarch provided one explanation why devotees may have favoured great *asclepieia* located outside the cities: 'Why is the shrine of Aesculapius

---

Pergamum was constructed about 3 km southwestwards of the city (McDonagh 1989, 222–225; Bean 1979, 58–59; Deubner 1938). The *asclepieion* in Lebena was built on a hill (Melfi 2007, 607). The *asclepieion* of Kos was built on a hill as well, around 4 km from the city of Koans, within a grove planted with cypresses (Martin and Metzger 1992, 79–80).

25. Proximity to water sources was a precondition for the establishment of the *asclepieia* (see Israelowich 2015, 117; see also Riethmüller 2005, I, 385–387; Renberg 2017, 150–154). The early Epidaurian *asclepieion* was built in a wooded valley near to a spring (Martin and Metzger 1992, 105–110). The *asclepieion* in Pergamum was built around a spring also in a small, wooded valley (McDonagh 1989, 222–225; Bean 1979, 58–59; Deubner 1938). The *asclepieion* in Lebena was constructed on the southern coast of Crete on a hill, which dominated the harbour (Melfi 2007, 607). The Koan *asclepieion* was built close to thermal waters (Martin and Metzger 1992, 79–80).

26. For example, in the *asclepieion* of Pergamum there were altars dedicated to Asclepius as well as to Hygeia, Epione and Artemis (Martin and Metzger 1992, 102).

27. For example, the chryselephantine cult statue of Asclepius, half the size of that of Olympian Zeus at Athens, was made by the Parian sculptor Thrasymedes and hosted in the temple of the Epidaurian *asclepieion* (Paus. *Descr. Graec.* II, 27, 2 = T. 630). A cult statue of Asclepius along with a statue of his daughter, Hygeia, was the centre of worship in the temple of the *asclepieion* of Lebena (Melfi 2007, 88–96).

28. On the *abaton* of the *asclepieia*, see, for example, Renberg 2017, 126–167.

29. In Epidaurus, for example, after the reconstruction of the sanctuary, the nearby spring was not adequate, and the first special structures to bring water to the site were constructed. These waterways received and distributed the water from the Apollo Maleatas' spring (Martin and Metzger 1992, 115; Riethmüller 2005, v. I, 229–240).

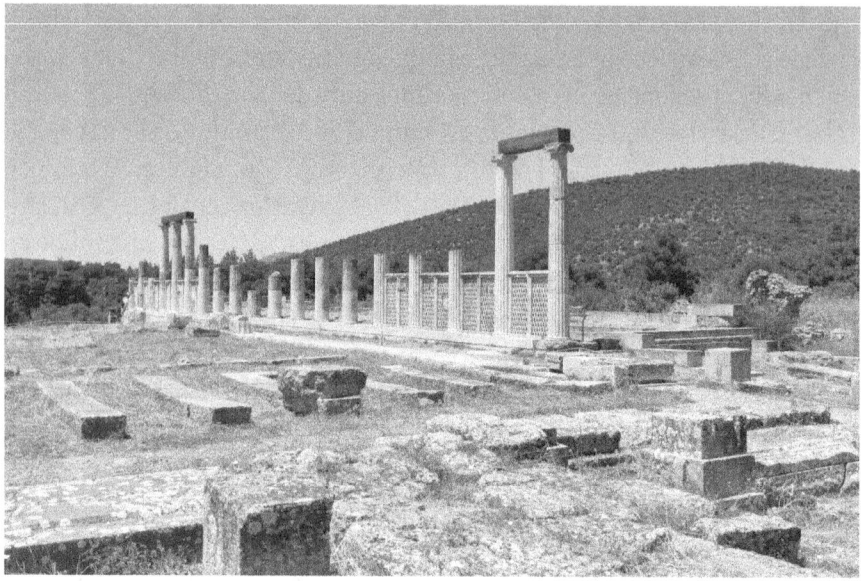

Figure 2 The stoa of *abaton* at the *asclepieion* of Epidaurus.

Source: George E. Koronaios, CC0, via Wikimedia Commons

outside the city? Is it because they considered it more healthful to spend their time outside the city than within its walls? In fact, the Greeks, as might be expected, have their shrines of Asclepius situated in places which are both clean and high...' (Plut. *Aet. Rom.* 94, 286 c–d, trans. Babbitt 1936).

The same attitude is expressed by Vitruvius, writing in the first century BCE, who argues that the temples of the god of medicine should be established in healthy surroundings:

> Finally, propriety will be due to natural causes if, for example, in the case of all sacred precincts we select very healthy neighbourhoods with suitable springs of water in the places where the fanes are to be built, particularly in the case of those to Aesculapius and to Health, gods by whose healing powers great numbers of the sick are apparently cured. For when their diseased bodies are transferred from an unhealthy to a healthy spot, and treated with waters from health-giving springs, they will the more speedily grow well. The result will be that the divinity will stand in higher esteem and find his dignity increased, all owing to the nature of his site.
> (Vitr. *De arch.* I, 2, 7, trans. Morgan 1914)

These observations of the ancient writers (see Baker 2017, 146–149) seem to be confirmed by modern research that investigates the impact of natural and urban settings on human health and well-being. In particular, the *asclepieia* can be seen as *therapeutic landscapes*, a term introduced by the health/medical geographer Wilbert Gesler in the early 1990s.[30]

Gesler (1992) describes the potential interrelation between health and certain places associated with treatment and healing (cf. Williams 1999; Khachatiurians 2006, 16; Velarde, Fryb and Tveitb 2007, 200). According to his definition, a landscape is perceived as therapeutic 'when physical and built environments, social conditions, and human perceptions combine to produce an atmosphere which is conducive to healing' (Gesler 1996, 95). The therapeutic character of some landscapes is amplified by their long-term reputation of healing and their connection with divine or miraculous healing interventions. Further, there might be local conditions which promote cures, like certain 'historical events, cultural beliefs, social relations and personal experiences' (Gesler 1996, 95). In his view, the term *landscape* does not refer to a certain kind of natural environment but is mostly a metaphorical perception of spatial areas that combine specific material conditions and symbolic meanings, and reflect particular values and perceptions (Gesler 1992, 743; Khachatiurians 2006, 19).

Asclepieia seemingly incorporated the major features of *therapeutic landscapes* as described by Gesler. Most of the sanctuaries were established in places which were perceived as sacred before the rise of the Asclepius cult (cf. Gesler 1992, 181; Edelstein and Edelstein 1998, v. II, 233). Apollo or other secondary healing deities had paved the way for the arrival of Asclepius to these sites.[31] The Epidaurian *asclepieion* was built in the wider region of Mount Kynortion, which had been devoted to healing deities since the prehistoric period (2800–1800 BCE). In the early seventh century, a sanctuary was built in honour of Apollo, who was named Maleatas after a local deity, and enjoyed worship for his healing powers (Martin and Metzger 1992, 105–110; Melfi 2010, 329). The first sanctuary of Asclepius in Pergamum was erected at the area where an unknown deity was previously worshipped (McDonagh 1989, 222–225; Bean 1979, 58–59; Deubner 1938). The *asclepieion* of Lebena was established at the site which previously belonged to Achelous or the Nymphs (Melfi 2009, 617; Nutton 2005, 106).

---

30. For a preliminary application of Gesler's theory to the Asclepius sanctuaries, see Panagiotidou 2013, 2021b.
31. Gesler (1993) in his case study on Epidaurus presents the main elements of *therapeutic landscapes* which are seen in the Epidaurian *asclepieion*. However, the same elements can be applied to the other great *asclepieia* as well; cf. Khachatiurians 2006, 50–52.

The Koan *asclepieion* was built in the sacred grove of Apollo Kyparissios (Martin and Metzger 1992, 79–80). Furthermore, various mythical traditions conveyed narratives about Asclepius and his superhuman healing powers, which were assumed to be more evident at the great healing centres. These stories formulated the wider conceptual context for the spread of Asclepius' reputation as a divine physician (cf. Gesler 1992, 178, 182; Panagiotidou 2013).

The isolation of the *asclepieia* from urban settings, and their situatedness in natural environments might have been conducive to recovery and well-being (see Christopoulou-Aletra, Togia and Varlami 2010; Baker 2017). Thousands of supplicants full of hope and expectations of healing departed from their home cities, and travelled short or long distances to the god's great sanctuaries.[32]

Although the cities of the Graeco-Roman world might not be comparable with modern metropolises, there certainly would still have been a continuous hustle and bustle, people would have been on the move and the construction works promoted by the Roman emperors would have affected ordinary urban life (White 1990, 26–30; Gesler 2003, 22; Israelowich 2015, 124–134). Thus, when the supplicants arrived at an Asclepius sanctuary, they entered a totally different environment, and might have had the feeling that they were in a place where health could be restored (see Christopoulou-Aletra, Togia and Varlami 2010; Baker 2017). The natural landscape of the sanctuaries with the holy springs and groves might have had an immediate effect, as the visitors felt released from the daily stressors of the cities (cf. Gesler 1993, 178–179; see Baker 2017). The enclosure of the *asclepieia* within the *temenos* might also have helped to enhance the Asclepius supplicants' 'sense of refuge and security' (Gesler 1993, 179; cf. Panagiotidou 2021a).

Maria Velarde and her colleagues (2007, 199, 210) have reviewed the existing literature focused on the health effects of viewing landscapes. Their research suggests that mere visual exposure to natural landscapes can be conducive to short-term relief from stress and mental fatigue, accelerate physical recovery, and offer long-term improvement of human health and well-being (cf. Christopoulou-Aletra, Togia and Varlami 2010; Baker 2017; Ulrich 1984, 1999). The short-term effects may include positive changes in blood pressure (cf. Ulrich 1981; Ulrich et al. 1991; Hartig

---

32. On the significance of sleeping in a particular place during incubation, see Patton 2004, 203–204.

et al. 2003; Ottosson and Grahn 2005; Lohr and Pearson-Mims 2006), heart rate (cf. Ulrich 1981; Heerwagen 1990; Ulrich et al. 1991; Laumann, Gärling and Stormark 2003; Ottosson and Grahn 2005), muscle tension (cf. Ulrich et al. 1991), and brain activity (cf. Ulrich 1981; Nakamura and Fujii 1992), which can be observed in less than five minutes after visual exposure to natural settings (Velarde, Fryb and Tveitb 2007, 210; cf. Ulrich 2002). Velarde's (2007) research indicates the significant role of water in these settings, a factor also noted by Gesler (1992, 1993, 182, 1998). As already mentioned, proximity to natural springs was one of the characteristics of the great *asclepieia*.

Although, it is doubtless that political motivations, financial interests, cultural preferences and social dynamics all played a role in the foundation and development of the Asclepius cult, and local conditions would, at least to some extent, have dictated the architectural design of the *asclepieia*, it seems that the main purpose of the Asclepius temples was to propagate the healing power of Asclepius. Every element of their natural settings and constructed environments was apparently dedicated to this purpose. The long-term reputation of *asclepieia* as healing centres, where treatments were achieved through divine interventions, attracted suffering persons who sought recovery (cf. Gesler 1992, 735–736). Meanwhile, the patients' beliefs in the divine healing powers of Asclepius and expectations of recovery following direct communication with the god, and their predispositions to believe in superhuman healing powers, meant that the *asclepieia* can be described as *Therapeutic Landscapes*: A place where cures and treatments might be possible through a kind of placebo effect (cf. Gesler 1993).

From Despair to Hope: From Doctors' Rejection to Asclepius Temples

In the wider conceptual context of the Graeco-Roman world, affliction by an illness or a disease would entail a violent disturbance of patients' lives and their organic balance, which threatened their survival and well-being (cf. Lasagna et al. 1954; Leventhal et al. 1982, 55–86). Since the origins and reasons of such afflictions were usually obscure and the duration of suffering was often unknown, with the prospect of chronic pain and death, the entailed uncertainty could hardly be tolerable and could be accompanied by further emotional (e.g. fear), cognitive (e.g. worry) and behavioural (e.g. inaction) implications (Carleton 2016a; cf. Freeston et al. 1994; Dugas, Gosselin and Ladouceur 2001, 552; Panagiotidou 2021b). In particular, the fear and anxiety which derives from the unknown development of an illness or a disease and its unknown consequences for the patient pertains to the elementary and universal *fear of the unknown*, which has its origins in the lack of knowledge and information about a perceived stimulus and is considered to be at the bottom of all kinds of fears experienced by humans (Carleton 2016a, 2016b; cf. Panagiotidou 2021a). Fear of the unknown and the so-called 'intolerance of uncertainty', when not developed into pathological disorders (e.g. depression), urge people to find ways to reduce these negative feelings and their possible implications. In this light, the people of Graeco-Roman antiquity would have experienced the infliction by an illness or a disease as a crucial turning point in their lives, which would have induced intense feelings of uncertainty and fear of the unknown.[33] The deep desire to relieve these negative feelings and to gain recovery would have urged patients to make decisions and to take actions in order to deal with their condition (Panagiotidou 2011, 129; cf. Dillon 1994, 239–240; Molen 2019, 1).

At that critical moment, a patient could consult a physician asking for treatment, resort to the temple of a healing deity or hero, visit an *asclepieion* or seek folk healers for help. The availability of all these healing alternatives was due to the medical pluralism of the era and offered a certain range of choices to patients (Wickkiser 2008, 42–44; see Oberhelman 2013; Israelowich 2015, 31, 46–51; Panagiotidou 2016c; cf. Aristid. *Or.* XLVIII, 31–35, XLVII, 57; *Anth. Pal.* VI, 330)

In particular, the growing presence of professional physicians in the wider environment of the Graeco-Roman cities made them a reasonable resort for people who experienced symptoms of illnesses.[34] People who saw others consulting doctors and heard stories about others' personal experiences with the art of medicine would have implicitly stored the consultation of doctors as a healing alternative in their memory systems, which they would have been able to appeal to, when faced with health

---

33. On the feelings of uncertainty and fear of the unknown that the supplicants of Asclepius might have experienced, see Panagiotidou 2021a, 2021b.
34. On the abundance of professional doctors – as well as of other kinds of healers – in the Graeco-Roman cities, see, for example, Nutton 2005, 152–155, 314; Israelowich 2015, 124–134.

problems (Panagiotidou 2016a, 85-86).³⁵ Through processes of cultural conditioning,³⁶ doctors formed a particular cultural category, i.e. that of medical experts who were members of the professional sector of medical care. Personal encounters with human doctors familiarized patients with the medical techniques and practices, and people gradually formed and shared common expectations of what medical professionalists could accomplish. In these settings, professional doctors' tendency to deny treatments to patients whom they diagnosed with chronic or fatal diseases and decided that they could not cure, would have entailed negative conditioning (see previous chapter; cf. Demand 1994, 45; Jouanna 1999, 110; Wickkiser 2008, 25, 118-119, notes 53 and 54; Renberg 2017, 23-24). That is not to say that negative conditioning led to a general devaluation of human doctors and medicine. It would rather entail the admission that doctors, who were considered to be authorities in the art of medicine because of their skills and knowledge, abided by the limits of medicine as a human art (see previous chapter).³⁷

In addition, given that health is one of the most sensitive domains of human life, people would have perceived doctors not only as professional experts in the medical art, but also as personal consultants and caretakers under whose protection they placed themselves and to whom they turned their hopes for recovery (Edelstein and Edelstein 1998, v. II, 111-112). Sick people probably were in need of a caring doctor who would be eager to listen to them with sympathy, and treat them wisely, possessing the appropriate means and skills to help them (cf. Welch 1972, 193; Blum 1985, 406). Therefore, for patients, who suffered from illnesses and diseases, a treatment rejection by doctors could prove shocking (Patton 2004, 198-199; Wickkiser 2008, 26; Renberg 2017, 23-24, 213-214). Essentially, a doctor's refusal to provide treatments and his negative attitude towards a disease or illness could reasonably be taken to mean that healing was actually impossible. Such an inference could demolish a patient's hope and belief in recovery, intensifying his or her feelings of uncertainty and fear of the unknown future, which could conceal chronic morbidity or

---

35. I examine the process of priming as the subliminal storing of information received from the perceivable surroundings in the mnemonic systems, more thoroughly in the following chapter.
36. Again, conditioning as a cognitive mode of cultural learning is more thoroughly examined in the next chapter.
37. Some preliminary ideas of this section presented at the XXI IAHR World Congress that took place in Erfurt, Germany, 23-29 August 2015; see also Panagiotidou 2016b, 15, 19.

even mortality. Those feelings of uncertainty and the fear of the unknown could transform a patient's need of hope into despair, inducing nocebo responses and leading him or her to depression, and ultimately death. In this way, the authoritative and otherwise protective figure of doctors operated as the external 'emotional trigger' which raised patients' feelings of anxiety and insecurity, probably reducing the impact of their own self-healing resources, and potentially worsening their clinical condition (cf. Kaptchuk, Miller and Colloca 2009, 531; Colloca et al. 2010).[38]

However, human beings have evolved a specific cognitive strategy of self-deception in order to react to vexatious and adverse conditions. According to Joseph Bulbulia (2006, 95), this tendency to self-deceive constitutes *an adaptive error*, which allows humans to adopt an optimistic attitude and strive to survive, even though the surrounding reality seems abysmal. Therefore, patients, who were rejected by human doctors, could not easily give up looking for healing alternatives. At this crucial moment, they would have looked for reasons to hope for recovery, even when such an outcome seemed impossible. And a visit to the temple of a healing god or hero would appear as a hopeful choice, which could save them from chronic suffering or even death (Panagiotidou 2011, 130).[39] Asclepius, in particular, would seem the most appropriate candidate for the role of a heroic saviour, since he was not just a healing deity, but was also a doctor himself (Ael. *Fr.* 89; *Anth. Pal.* VI, 330; Edelstein and Edelstein 1998, v. II, 169; Wickkiser 2008, 32–33; Csepregi 2011; Renberg 2017, 215). The deified physician was the peoples' patron who cared about their needs and personal affairs (cf. Błaśkiewicz 2014). People might feel safe in his hands, taking refuge in his sanctuaries (Edelstein and Edelstein 1998, v. II, 111–113). Asclepius, meanwhile, was thought to be eager to help them, and even thought to have cured patients who did not believe in his power:

> Ambrosia from Athens, blind in one eye. She came as a supplicant to the god. Walking about the sanctuary, she ridiculed some of the cures as being unlikely and impossible, the lame and the blind becoming well from only seeing a dream. Sleeping here, she saw a vision. It seemed to her the god

---

38. On the significance of the doctor–patient interrelation in clinical contexts, see Blum 1985, 403; Monroe, Holleman and Holleman 1992; Brody 2000; Humphrey 2002, 274; Kaptchuk 2002; Benedetti et al. 2007.

39. On the reasons for which patients, suffering mainly from chronic diseases and negative conditioning in scientific medicine, resort to traditional healing methods, see Kaptchuk 2002, 818, and further Zollman and Vickers 1999.

came to her and said he would make her well, but she would have to pay a fee by dedicating a silver pig in the sanctuary as a memorial of her ignorance. When he had said these things, he cut her sick eye and poured a medicine over it. When day came she left well.

(*IG* II(2), 1, 121, IV, trans. LiDonnici 1995, A4)

This story describes the possible reactions of patients who would have read or heard of the miraculous healing narratives conveyed in the inscriptions and could have disputed the possibility of healing. Even if the story of Ambrosia was fictitious, this story served a rhetorical purpose: it was displayed to convince visitors of the immense healing power of Asclepius and his willingness to help even those who would have disputed his superhuman healing powers. The supposed message of Asclepius to his supplicants was indirect but clear: 'You can be surprised and dispute my healing powers. In any case, I am eager to treat you'.

Further, ancient sources explicitly mention cases in which patients, who had despaired of (or been rejected by) their human doctors, turned their hopes to Asclepius in order to receive a cure. The thank-offering of Aeschines the Orator to Asclepius is exemplary:[40] 'Despairing of human art, and placing all my hope in the Divinity, I left Athens, mother of beautiful children, and was cured in three months, Asklepios, by coming to thy grove, of an ulcer on my head that had continued for a year' (*Anth. Graec.* VI, 330, trans. Paton 1916,).

In this view, faith in the superhuman healing power of Asclepius could be a form of *adaptive error* which provided patients with reasons to hope and believe that they could disprove – through divine intervention – the bleak prognoses given by doctors, who were restrained by their own human nature. Thus, the Asclepius cult could operate as a placebo system, that intervened to cover the gaps left, when physical and natural procedures failed to bring relief and well-being (cf. Bulbulia 2006, 103; cf. Ael. *Fr.* 89 = T. 399; 100 = T. 321, 405; *Anth. Pal.* VI, 330 = T. 404; M. Ant. *In Sem. Ips.* V, 8 = T. 407). And in the case of the Asclepius temples, religious healing was interwoven with medical procedures, giving the perception that these were places where treatments and cures were feasible.[41]

---

40. Cf. *IG* XIV, no. 966 = T. 438 as well as the case of Aelius Aristides who turned to Asclepius, after being disappointed by human doctors' failure to relieve him from his illness (see Downie 2013a, 90; Renberg 2017, 23–24, 26, esp. n. 70; Panagiotidou 2021b).

41. On the association and similarities between doctors' medical practices and temple medicine exerted at the *asclepieia*, see Israelowich 2015, 46, 52–62.

That is not to say that there was a universal pattern according to which people first consulted a doctor and afterwards resorted to Asclepius. As shown in the previous chapter, the medical pluralism of Graeco-Roman life provided many healing options pertaining to professional, folk and popular domains, that people could make use of depending on their personal attitudes towards various health providers, on the availability of the latter in patients' surroundings and on circumstances. In any case, the original motivation for those people who turn to Asclepius for healing was probably the desire for life and well-being.

Believing What Others Tend to Believe: Asclepius as the Supreme Authority

Beyond the *asclepieia*, Asclepius' representations and symbols were present almost everywhere in the wider settings of Graeco-Roman cities. Coins bearing the image of the god were minted in Epidaurus and other cities, advertising his particular bonds with these regions.[42] Votive plaques and statues representing Asclepius and his worshippers were set up in many places within cities, propagating his superhuman medical skills.[43] Literary sources also mention Asclepius, indicating that his cult was widely known among his contemporaries (Wickkiser 2008, 38; see Aeschin. *In Ctes.* 66–67 = T. 566; Apul. *Flor.* 18 = T. 608; *Apol.* 55 = T. 609; Arist. *Res Publ. Athen.* 56.4 = T. 567; August. *De civ. D.* III, 17 = T. 507; Herond. *Mim.* IV, 1–95 = T. 482; Iambl. *VP* 27, 126 = T. 487, 842; Paus. *Descr. Graec.* II, 27, 6 = T. 488; Pl. *Ion* 530A = T. 560; Xen. *Mem.* III, 13, 3 = T. 723; Q. Ser. Sammon. *Lib. Medicin. Prooem.*, 1–10 = T. 615; Theoc. *Epigr.* VII = T. 501; Theophr. *Char.* XXI, 10 = T. 542; etc.). Particularly the comedies of Greek playwrights Aristophanes (*Plut.*, 633–747 = T. 421) and Menander (*P. Didot.* b, 1–15 = T. 419) and of Roman Plautus (*Curc.* 216–273 = T. 430) refer to Asclepius and his sanctuaries – references

---

42. For example, coins from Epidaurus depicted Asclepius on the obverse, and a cupping instrument on the reverse. Bronze coins from Pergamum in Mysia bore Asclepius' head on the obverse, and the *caduceus* on the reverse. Coins from Trikka, probably depicting Asclepius, intended to link him to this city and to neighbouring Larisa. As we have seen, the city of Kos minted coins with the head of Hippocrates on the one side, and the staff and snake of Asclepius on the other; Wickkiser 2008, 1, 36, 49, 55, 56, 132; Hart 2000, 11–12. For a detailed presentation of the ancient coins related to medicine and Asclepius, see Hart 1966.
43. Even in Rome, sculptural and relief representations of Asclepius indicate his prominent presence in the city; see Renberg 2006/2007, 120.

which suggest that audiences were familiar with Asclepius and the healing of diseases at his sanctuaries (Wickkiser 2008, 38; Panagiotidou 2013, 2016c). In addition, swearing by Asclepius implies that people respected the divine physician (Men. *Boeot.* Fr. 91 = T. 618; *Sam.* 94–95 = T. 619; Gal. *De Comp. Medic. Sec. Loc.* Cp. 3 [XIII, 271–272] = T. 620; Julian. *Heracl. Cynic.* 234 D = T. 621; Stat. *Silv.* III, *Praef.* = T. 550; Theoph. *Ad Autol.* III, 2 = T. 622).

The transmission of the ideas and precepts about Asclepius through material and verbal signs – based on the human ability for symbolic communication – provided a representational context in which social information about the god's healing power flowed, and was shared by people of the Graeco-Roman world (Panagiotidou 2013, 2016c).

Through social interaction and various cognitive processes (Roepstorff, Niewöhner and Beck 2010, 1057),[44] humans are able to learn from others. As I briefly implied in the previous section, even just the observation of others' behaviours and choices can provide information about the value of certain objects, artefacts, places, actions or even other people,[45] affecting the way in which people reflect on themselves, others, and the world as well as the practices they follow (Frith and Frith 2012, 289).

Social learning draws on multiple learning mechanisms (including conditioning and instrumental learning) and shares the same neural systems with the non-social reward-based learning, in which values are represented in the ventromedial prefrontal cortex and reward expectations are represented in the ventral striatum (Frith and Frith 2012, 293; see further Schultz 2006; Lin, Adolphs and Rangel 2012). The same reward learning system is also activated when people observe others approaching or avoiding certain places (Campbell-Meiklejohn et al. 2010; Frith and Frith 2012, 293; cf. Panagiotidou 2016c, 2021a). In this way, social learning mediates through the ascription of values to specific places and objects (Siegel 2002; Schultz 2008; Frith and Frith 2012, 289). In particular, individuals tend to attribute higher value to places which are visited by many people than to those places that are less popular (Frith and Frith 2012, 293).

On a sensorial level, it is difficult to evaluate information about a certain object or place. People, therefore, try to draw inferences about these

---

44. On the perceptual and rational associations between external conditions and events, and representations of the world in the human mind, see Shanks 2010.
45. On social learning through observation of other people's behaviour, and its significance for placebo responses, see Bootzin and Caspi 2002; Iacoboni 2009; Colloca and Benedetti 2009; Mazzoni et al. 2010.

through information in their surroundings. Congruity between individual and normative opinions modifies activity in the ventral striatum in a manner similar to dopamine-mediated reward signals, which appear in the same brain regions during reinforcement learning. The ventral striatum updates values via inputs from the hippocampus, amygdala, frontal cortex, and the mesolimbic dopamine pathway (Figure 3). Especially the dopamine system seems to mediate social influences on valuation, since 'it signals the magnitude of reward relative to what is expected' from acquiring a certain object or visiting a specific place 'rather than on some absolute scale' (Campbell-Meiklejohn et al. 2010, 1168; cf. Schultz 2006).

Thus, when people of the Graeco-Roman world observed others visiting the Asclepius sanctuaries and being cured of their ailments, dopaminergic signals in their brains could perhaps have carried information about the reward's magnitude, and increased their expectations of visiting the same places and participating in the same practices (Panagiotidou 2016c, 2021a; cf. Campbell-Meiklejohn et al. 2010, 1168).

Furthermore, opinions formulated by experts might also influence the evaluation of objects, places and practices, since they 'provide a source of prior information' about these matters which is available and might bias the general view (Campbell-Meiklejohn et al. 2010, 1168). This bias is enforced by pre-established beliefs about the experts' opinions as valid indications of the objects' values. Experts are considered to be persons who know the non-social features of specific objects, places and

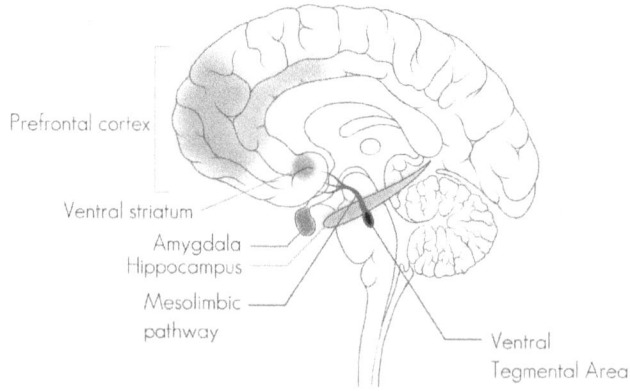

Figure 3 The brain: reward system and social learning.

Source: Patrick J. Lynch, medical illustrator C. Carl Jaffe, MD, cardiologist FvasconcellosWhidou, CC BY-SA 4.0, https://creativecommons.org/licenses/by-sa/4.0, via Wikimedia Commons

practices. Thus, their opinions, judgments and suggestions might influence people's reward expectations concerning the acquirement of a certain object, or visiting a specific place or following a particular practice (Campbell-Meiklejohn et al. 2010, 1168–1169; cf. Panagiotidou 2016c; see also Henrich 2015, 117–139). Especially in conditions of uncertainty and despair, people's tendency to believe what others, and especially respected people, tend to believe constitutes a common human heuristic (Bulbulia 2006, 93; cf. Panagiotidou 2016c, 2021a).

Particularly, in the Graeco-Roman world, doctors were perceived as health experts, who enjoyed the respect of other people because of their skills in the treatment and healing of illnesses and diseases (Wickkiser 2008, 10–12). Asclepius' authority, however, was greater than that of the physicians because of his divine nature, medical profession, ubiquity, and omnipotence, but also because of his permanent disposition and benevolent eagerness to heal anyone asking for his help. The acknowledgement of Asclepius as superior doctor by other physicians increased the god's reputation, and thereby people's reward expectations. These expectations would have been further reinforced, when patients observed other people visiting his temples and receiving treatments.

In this way, patients could use other people's reactions – pertaining to folk sector medical healing options – when they faced health problems, as well as doctors' suggestions – who comprised the professional sector – in order to determine healing alternatives available to them. Others' opinions about the effectiveness of Asclepius' healing powers would have wielded strong social influences on patients' brain systems followed by direct alternations in their valuation systems. We can surmise that this social influence would to a great extent contribute to the rapid spread of knowledge about Asclepius and his rise in popularity in the Graeco-Roman world.

Continual interaction between other agents' actions, expert's opinions, material representations, verbal expressions, social norms, precepts and beliefs about the Asclepius cult would have mediated the development of a visit to the god's temples into a specific pattern of practice. This practice would have been an alternative therapeutic choice in people's minds and brains as well as in the external world. Therefore, the event of a person's affliction by a disease would have interacted with the 'context-dependent, higher-order model' of the Asclepius cult, which would have framed single individual events in terms of other people's prior experiences (cf. Roepstorff, Niewöhner and Beck 2010, 1056–1057; Panagiotidou 2013).

Chapter 4

Taking the Journey

Arriving at the *Asclepieia*

So far, I have provided some insights into how people of the Graeco-Roman world, through a combination of personal reflections, social interactions and multiple learning mechanisms, could have formulated specific ideas and conceptions about Asclepius and his healing powers as well as about other healing options provided in their cultural surroundings.[1] In this framework, I presented Asclepian medicine as part of the wider medical pluralism of the Graeco-Roman era that provided various but not mutually exclusive choices – consulting folk healers, professional doctors, healing deities, etc. – which people could make when confronted by health problems. In this chapter, I examine how particular influences and motivations, common in people's social and cultural surroundings, would have mediated patients' decisions to visit an Asclepius sanctuary, and, further, how the particular context of the *asclepieia* could have influenced supplicants' personal perceptions, conceptions, feelings, and expectations for healing and established appropriate conditions for the activation of placebo effects.

In this framework, the healing inscriptions and anatomical votive offerings displayed in the *asclepieia* are not taken as proofs of real cures that the dedicators actually experienced. I mainly consider the healing narratives and anatomical *ex votos* as a major means used by the cult to advertise Asclepius' healing powers, to predict supplicants' reactions and possible

---

1. Quinton Deeley argues 'the process whereby individuals acquire conceptions, motivations, and behaviours that are typical of their social group' as 'enculturation' and suggests that this can be explained by 'a conjunction of social referencing, mentalizing, and associative learning' (2004, 255).

suspicion of the prospect of miraculous interventions, and to convince new-comers of the possibility of experiencing a divine cure during incubation (see, for example, Schörner 2015, 409). In this light, I examine the possible cognitive processes that would have mediated the interpretation of the recorded events in the cult context and would have framed patients' individual needs and expectations of relief and recovery conducive to placebo responses.

Therefore, I do not intend to prove that the healing narratives reported in the inscriptions could have actually happened through the operation of placebo effects. Many illnesses and diseases (e.g. sterility problems, ulcers, gout, headache, insomnia) described in these narratives could be treated through the activation of placebo responses. However, clearly there are cases in which placebo effect would not be enough to bring recovery (e.g. prolonged pregnancies, mutilations, etc.). Although we cannot exclude the possibility of some supplicants to have had actual healing experiences in the sanctuaries and to have made such dedications, the public exposure to the healing inscriptions and anatomical votive offerings was a crucial component of the wider religious environment of the *asclepieia* that intended to influence and manipulate supplicants' thoughts, emotions and expectations of healing, thus contributing to placebo responses.

Hope as Motivational Force: Planning the Journey to *Asclepieion*

In the Graeco-Roman world, people afflicted by an illness or a disease could make the decision to consult a professional doctor, ask the aid of a folk healer, evoke a healing deity or visit one of the Asclepius temples. In seeking recovery, a patient could make whatever choice he or she would like. The same person could make use of all the available healing options, in whatever order, or to choose one or more of them. In any case, the motivational force of personal decisions would have been the hope for relief and recovery (cf. Panagiotidou 2021b). Charles Snyder and his colleagues (2000, 747) define hope as 'the perceived capability to derive pathways to desired goals and motivate oneself via agentic thinking to initiate and sustain movement along those pathways'. According to their hope theory, agency and pathways are two interrelated and requisite components of hope (Snyder et al. 2000, 748). In particular, *goals* are the 'anchors of hope' since they are inherent in any kind of planned activity, and motivate behaviour (Snyder et al. 2000, 748). In order for people to carry out a movement or action, they should 'believe that they are able to generate workable routes to their goals' (Snyder et al. 2000, 749). This self-conviction, which motivates people to move along an imagined pathway toward their target-destination, is defined as *agency* (Snyder et al. 2000, 749).

In the Asclepius case, patients were motivated by their goal to recover (Panagiotidou 2021b). Their perceptual ability allowed them to imagine pathways towards this goal. A first possible course for them was to visit and consult a human doctor.[2] However, when the human medical skill had proven to be ineffective without offering any chance for recovery, positive *agentic thinking* would have allowed patients to envision alternative pathways to retain their hope (cf. Snyder et al. 2000, 749). Supporting this view, modern scientific evidence indicates that high-hope people tend to perceive themselves as able to imagine and generate new routes, when the initial course seems to be blocked (Snyder et al. 2000, 749; see further Snyder et al. 1991; Snyder 1994; Irving, Snyder and Crowson 1998). Thus, in the Graeco-Roman context, visiting an Asclepius temple would have been perceived of as a pathway to healing, among other pathways that were known in their cultural surroundings and that could lead to cure. The choice to follow this pathway derived from the person's learning history and from previous healing experiences in the Asclepius temples as testified by other members of his or her social group.

In this light, the decision itself of visiting an Asclepius sanctuary could increase people's hopes (cf. Snyder et al. 2000, 755).[3] Although patients could feel disillusioned from suffering or from a physicians' refusal to help them or from the failure of an applied treatment, the fact that they had another option and could implement another pathway toward the goal of recovery could raise agentic thoughts. Furthermore, modern research suggests that patients are able to experience an improvement in their condition upon reaching the decision to follow a specific treatment, even

---

2. I should note once again that this script of actions was not canonical, and visiting an *asclepieion* did not necessarily presuppose that patients had previously consulted a doctor or experienced a rejection by human physicians. On the contrary, as shown in the previous chapters, various alternative scenarios and pathways to healing were available and would have been appropriated by individuals in response to their occasional needs depending on their current capabilities and options.

3. P. M. Morris (1982) examined a group of patients who decided to visit the Church of Our Lady in Lourdes. His findings show a significant decrease of patients' anxiety and depression upon their decision to visit the church.

before this treatment actually begins (Snyder et al. 2000, 757; Constantino et al. 2011, 185; cf. Morris 1982; Beckham 1989) – reflecting a kind of placebo effect. Consistently, patients who travelled short or long distances to *asclepieia* could experience a revival of hope (both pathways and agency thoughts) and symptoms of relief upon their decision to undertake the journey. However, this initial improvement would not last for long, if there was no further evidence indicating that the recently followed pathway was workable (cf. Snyder et al. 2000, 757).

Inducing Expectations: Arriving at the Asclepius Sanctuary

Patients, travelling to the Asclepius temples, would have probably been preoccupied with their own illnesses (diseases or sickness), full of hopes of a cure. Their hopes and excitement could possibly be aroused upon their arrival at the sanctuary (Edelstein and Edelstein 1998, v. II, 161; Tick 2001, 248; Panagiotidou 2011, 132; Cilliers and Retief 2013, 86).

The whole environment and structure of the *asclepieia* tended to induce and manipulate patients' expectations of their on-coming healing. In particular, therapy outcome expectations are defined as 'cognitions regarding a probable future resulting from treatment' (Constantino et al. 2011, 186). This kind of expectation can be inspired by the personal history of the patient and his or her interrelation with the health provider and other people as well as by their common experiences and the general context in which healing procedures take place (Oken 2008, 2814). Although there are no detailed descriptions of the daily life at the Asclepius sanctuaries, indirect references in literary sources along with the arrangement of the dedications in the *temenos* give us some sense of the whole atmosphere and the probable human interactions within the Asclepius cult settings.

The most graphic description is indirectly outlined in Herondas's *Mimiambi* (IV, 1–95 = T. 482), dated in the mid-third century BCE (see Versnel 1981, 63; Dillon 1994, 255; Edelstein and Edelstein 1998, v. II, 188–190; Chamoux 2003, 335–336; Ferguson 2003, 176; Dignas 2007, 169–170). This work dramatizes the visit of two women possibly to the *asclepieion* of Kos. The heroine Cynno along with her friend and at least one of her slaves arrived at the sanctuary early in the morning. She wanted to offer a sacrifice to Asclepius, who had cured her disease with his 'gentle hands'.[4] Hailing the god and his divine relatives, Cynno offered a cock and a votive tablet, which she deposited next to the cult image of Hygeia that stood close to one of the altars in the holy precinct. The company admired the inscribed votive offerings which adorned the *temenos*. Cynno ordered her slave to go and call the *sacristan* in order to open the gates of the temple. She would like to show her friend even more beautiful things than she had ever seen in her whole life. However, her order was meaningless, since the doors were already open, and the visitors could enter the temple. They went inside, and while they were admiring the exhibited unique pieces of art, the *sacristan* approached and became involved in a discussion with them. He assured Cynno that her sacrifice was entirely favourable to the god. Cynno defended herself for the small price of her offering and promised to come back again along with her husband and children bringing larger offerings. She recommended her friend to 'remember to carve the leg of the fowl off carefully and give it to the *sacristan*, and put the mess into the mouth of the snake reverently, and souse the meat-offering' (Herond. *Mim.* IV, 88–92, trans. Knox 1922,). The *sacristan* also asked some of the holy bread; for the loss of this [?] was more serious to holy men than the loss of their portion' (Herond. *Mim.* IV, 94–95, trans. Knox 1922,) (Figure 4).

Herondas's *Mimiambos* IV offers a glimpse into the everyday life at the Koan *asclepieion*, as it might have been at least from the third century BCE to the end of Graeco-Roman antiquity. Despite potential local variations, the pattern can be outlined according to Herondas's description and other testimonies. Supplicants used to visit the *asclepieia* in order to pray for their family's well-being and their own good health.[5] Thus, *asclepieia* were much-frequented places, attracting both healthy and sick persons who might have been accompanied by their friends, relatives, and slaves. Entering the peaceful, natural environment of the sanctuaries, the visitors could *view* and be enchanted by the beauty of the landscape along with

---

4. Herond. *Mim.* IV, 16–18: 'be paying the price of cure from diseases that thou didst wipe away, Lord, by laying on us thy gentle hands' (trans. Knox 1922).
5. Marcus Aurelius, for instance, called for the aid of the healing deities, and intended to visit 'that spot where the god who is invested with the power may the more readily near' (Fronto, *Ep.* III, 9, 1–2 = T. 577). He would like to climb the hill of Pergamum where the Asclepius temple was located, and pray for his master's health (Edelstein and Edelstein 1998, v. II, 182; Renberg 2006/2007, 125). Beyond Marcus Aurelius, as noted in the previous chapter, many other supplicants probably visited the Asclepius temples for the same purpose (Edelstein and Edelstein 1998, v. II, 182; Renberg 2006/2007, 125; Dignas 2007, 170).

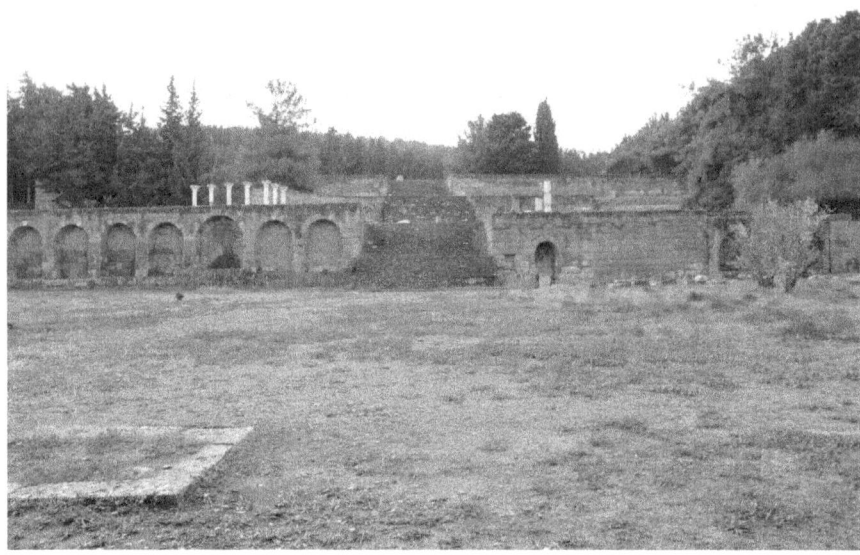

Figure 4 The *asclepieion* of Kos.

Source: Asurnipal, CC BY-SA 4.0, https://creativecommons.org/licenses/by-sa/4.0, via Wikimedia Commons

the shapeliness of the temple and other buildings which were decorated with unique masterpieces of art (cf. 'therapeutic landscapes'; Gesler 1992; Christopoulou-Aletra, Togia and Varlami 2010). They were allowed to walk around in the sanctuary admiring the thank-offerings exhibited in the precinct as well as within the temple. They could also meet people making dedications to the god's statues claiming that they had been healed, while they themselves could dedicate small offerings next to lavish dedications and pieces of art which adorned the sanctuaries (see, for example, Dillon 1994, 254–255; Dignas 2007, 169–170; Cilliers and Retief 2013, 75, 81–82; Mattern 2013, 24–25).

In addition, the supplicants could pray and observe others offer prayers and sacrifices to the god, hoping to be cured. Among the cult statues in the holy precinct, were altars in front of which supplicants spoke prayers of gratitude[6] to the divine physician. The form and the content of the prayers varied from extensive entreaties to simple, kind appeals to the

---

6. On prayers of gratitude in Greek antiquity, see Versnel 1981, 42–62.

god.[7] The supplicants prayed either in upright position or in prostration, probably hoping to influence the god through their posture.[8] The Romans, in particular, approached Asclepius with their heads covered according to their own fashion, although the rituals in the Roman *asclepieia* followed the Greek pattern.[9]

The altars were full of sacrifices and other offerings, including cakes with honey, cheese, and other foodstuffs (see Von Ehrenheim 2015, 49-73). The visitors could *smell* the odours of the sacrificial animals, which included cocks, pigs and oxen with local variations.[10] The offerings were probably given to the *sacristans* who would opine whether the sacrifice had been accepted or the supplicants should pray again. After the sacrifice was favoured by the god, the *sacristan* received his share of the offering, while another portion was given to the mouth of the sacred serpent. According to Herondas, the supplicants could take their portions back to their home and consume them there, while they also received some sacred bread to take with them as a means of protection.[11] This was perhaps the custom in

---

7. Arnobius (*Adv. Nat.* I, 49 = T. 576a, 584) comments the extensive entreaties which were full of piteous oaths and vows; Proclus, on the other hand, chose to pray to Asclepius in the old, gentle fashion of ancient Athenians (Marin. *Vit. Procl.*, Cp. 29 = T. 582, 728); Edelstein and Edelstein 1998, v. II, 184-185; on prayers, see Versnel 1981, esp. 25, 34-35, 51-56; Von Ehrenheim 2015, 73-74.

8. In the fourth century BCE, Diogenes the Cynic (*V Philosoph.* VI, 37-38) rejected the prostration and 'dedicated to Asclepius a bruiser who, whenever people fell on their faces, used to run up to them and beat them up' (trans. Hicks,); see also Edelstein and Edelstein 1998, v. II, 185.

9. Plaut. *Curc.* III, 389-390: 'Who's this that with covered head is saluting Æsculapius?' (trans. Riley 1912); see also Edelstein and Edelstein 1998, v. II 185.

10. In Cyrene, for example, goats were offered, a sacrifice which was forbidden in Epidaurus; Paus. *Descr. Graec.* II, 26, 09: 'There is this difference between the Cyreneans and the Epidaurians, that whereas the former sacrifice goats, it is against the custom of the Epidaurians to do so' (trans. Jones and Ormerod 1918). Although cocks are not mentioned in the Epidaurian *iamata*, they would have been a common sort of thank-offering affordable even for poorer supplicants (e.g. Socrates vowed a cock to Asclepius, and he ordered the accomplishment of his debt before he dies; Pl. *Phd.* 118A = T. 524; Lucian, *Bis Accus.* 5 = T. 525; Olympiod. *Pl. Phd. Comm.* p. 205, 24 = T. 526, p. 244, 17 = T. 527; Tert. *Apol.* XLVI, 5 = T. 528; Lactant. *Div. inst.* III, 20, 16-17 = T. 529; Lactant. *Inst. Epit.* 32, 4-5 = T. 530; cf. Artem. *Oneirocr.* V, 9 = T. 523; see, for example, Van Straten 1981, 68; Dillon 1994, 254-255; Edelstein and Edelstein 1998, v.II, 189-190; Von Ehrenheim 2015, 128-132).

11. Herond. *Mim.* IV, 94-95: 'The rest we will eat at home; and remember to take it away' (trans. Knox 1922).

Kos, while in other sanctuaries, like in Epidaurus, the supplicants should consume their shares from the sacrifices inside the holy precinct.[12]

Beyond individual prayers and sacrifices, the visitors could also attend the ordinary rituals which took place in the *asclepieia*. These observances were regularly held at least twice a day, in the morning and at nightfall.[13] The priests of Asclepius, usually wearing white clothes,[14] offered sacrifices upon the altars, while praying to the god.[15] Songs and hymns were sung during the ordinary rituals by the congregation or choirs sometimes comprised by slaves.[16] Paean was the most representative choral hymn chanted in honour of Asclepius with cithara accompaniment.[17]

One or more *sacristan*s oversaw the daily rituals, helped the priests in their duties, and perhaps guided the supplicants who were going to incubate in the *abaton*.[18] Although there are not enough literary sources about the administration of the great sanctuaries and the exact interplay between the priesthood, the temple servants, and the visitors, there might be personal communication among the *sacristan*s and supplicants who possibly received instructions about appropriate behaviour and actions within the *temenos* (Cilliers and Retief 2013, 81; Dignas 2007, 170).

In addition to the daily services and rituals performed by the Asclepian priesthood, and the offerings made by visitors who flocked to the great *asclepieia* every day, there were also public festivals which were repeated at certain intervals. These festivals varied in terms of their date and

---

12. Paus. *Descr. Graec.* II, 27, 1: 'All the offerings, whether the offerer be one of the Epidaurians themselves or a stranger, are entirely consumed within the bounds. At Titane too, I know, there is the same rule' (trans. Jones and Ormerod 1918).
13. These temple services were customary in the late Hellenistic and Roman period, although it is not known how often they were held in earlier centuries; Edelstein and Edelstein 1998, v. II, 193.
14. In the Pergamene *asclepieion*, the priests wore purple tunics (Tert. *De pall.* I, 1-2 = T. 492); on general regulations of clothing during Greek antiquity, see Mills 1984.
15. On the possible roles of the priests in the healing processes at the *asclepieia*, see, for example, Burnett 2015.
16. Certain songs were sung in the Epidaurian *asclepieion* in the morning; *Epigr. Graec.* 1027 = T. 598; see Edelstein and Edelstein 1998, v. II, 193-194, and esp. note 10.
17. Originally the *paean* was dedicated to Apollo; on the hymns and sermons in honour of Asclepius, see Edelstein and Edelstein 1998, v. II, 199-208; Ferguson 2003, 181-182. The verses of two *paean*s - only one of which is readable - devoted to Apollo and Asclepius have been found on an inscription from Erythrae of Ionia; see Bremmer 1981, 207-210.
18. Great sanctuaries, like this in Pergamum, usually had two *sacristan*s (Aristid. *Or.* XLVIII, 29 = T. 495).

frequency during the year in different regions.[19] However, the general pattern determined that the supplicants[20] met in the centre of the city, and from there went in procession to the temple, singing paeans in the god's honour. Upon their arrival at the sanctuary, they offered sacrifices[21] to Asclepius, a representation (a puppet) of whom[22] was seated on a couch.[23]

Most of the festivals were further accompanied by games, which were part of the cult and attracted many visitors from near and far in order to participate in or just attend to the competitions.[24] These games included gymnastics and, in some cases, music contests. Dramatic plays were regularly performed in the *asclepieia*. Although there are no literary sources about the theatrical works which were presented in the sanctuaries of Epidaurus, Pergamum, and Kos, both tragedies and comedies would have been dramatized, inspired by the myth, life and deeds of Asclepius (Edelstein and Edelstein 1998, v. II, 211).

In this wider cult context, patients entering the Asclepius sanctuary were bombarded by multiple contextual stimuli that triggered all their senses and could induce expectations of healing (Panagiotidou 2013, 2016c, 2021a). The aesthetic perception of the cult surroundings might enhance patients' subsequent religious experiences. Beyond the natural landscape

---

19. Some cities held the Asclepius festivals in spring (Aristid. *Or.* XLVIII, 74 = T. 570) and others in autumn (Philostr. *VA* IV). Some cities celebrated the god once (Cic. *Verr.* IV, 57, 127–128 = T. 554) and others twice a year (*CIG*, II, Add. no. 3641b); on the dates and frequency of the festivals, see also Edelstein and Edelstein 1998, v. II, 195–196.

20. There were also variations regarding the participants in these processions. In some cases, men, women and even young children could participate in the festivals (*IG* XII 9, 194 = T. 787), while in other celebrations, only men were allowed to take part (*IG* IV(2), 1, 128, I, 1–ii, 26 = T. 296). In the annual festival on Kos, the *Asclepiades* made themselves a lavish procession (Hippoc. *Ep.* 11, IX, p. 324–326 L = T. 568); on the participants to these festivals, see Edelstein and Edelstein 1998, v. II, 196.

21. The offerings varied from place to place and from time to time (Edelstein and Edelstein 1998, v. II, 197).

22. In early times, the devotees believed that Asclepius participated in the festivals and there was no need for the symbolic representation of his presence. The custom to place a puppet that was perceived as the embodiment of the god, upon a couch is dated in later centuries (Edelstein and Edelstein 1998, v. II, 197).

23. On the festivals in honour of Asclepius, see, for example, Edelstein and Edelstein 1998, v. II, 195–199; Wells 1998, 19–20.

24. The Epidaurian Games, for instance, were held every five years at least from the fifth century BCE onwards, and gradually acquired pan-Hellenistic reputation; Schol. in Pind., *Ad Nemeas*, V. 94b = T. 558, III, 147 = T. 559; Wells 1998, 19–20; on the games in honour of Asclepius, see Edelstein and Edelstein 1998, v. II, 208–213.

and architectural arrangement of the sanctuaries (see Chapter 3), the healing inscriptions displayed in various places within the *temenos*, recorded stories about people who had visited the *asclepieia* in the past and asked for divine cure (Panagiotidou 2013; see Dillon 1994, 240, 257–259). These stories would have circulated among the supplicants, who likely discussed with each other and the temple *sacristan*s about other people's previous healing experiences at the temples. The anatomical votive offerings were displayed as fragments of the healing experiences and narratives of persons who, suffering from various diseases, visited *asclepieia* and received divine cure.[25] This supposed biographical evidence was explicit testimonies of Asclepius' healing powers and intended to confirm the credibility of the divine treatments and to enhance the supplicants' expectations about positive health outcomes (see Dillon 1994, 257; Cilliers and Retief 2013, 75; cf. Constantino et al. 2011, 185). In this way, information flowing in the wider context would have influenced the patient's expectations and anticipations about recovery.

According to Albert Bandura, expectations can be classified in two categories: *outcome expectations*, characterized by the belief that certain actions will have certain outcomes, and *self-efficacy expectations*, based on the conviction that someone can successfully perform the appropriate actions in order to attain a desired result (Crow et al. 1999, 4; see Bandura 1997). In the Asclepius temples, supplicants were informed about the specific actions, rituals and purifications as well as about the process of incubation which they should follow in order to have personal communication with the god and divine treatment. They could also *see* other people following the same steps. In addition, they *heard* stories about the successful outcomes of these procedures. At least the literate persons could also read the stories written on the inscriptions. In this light, evidence about others' successful performances and curative experiences (e.g. seeing others succeeding), relative verbal attestations as well as patients' empathy and psychological states (hope, desire for relief) (Crow et al. 1999, 4) could enhance patients' expectations about both the treatment outcome and their own abilities to carry out the necessary actions in order to be cured.

---

25. Günther Schörner (2015, 399) has proposed a distinction between 'anatomical ex votos' which represent body parts dedicated in a ritual context associated with healing, and other 'body part votives' devoted for other purposes and in different contexts; on the problems of definition of the anatomical votive offerings, see Schörner 2015, 397–399.

According to Humphrey (see Chapter 1), a patient's expectation that following a particular treatment he or she is going to feel better, constitutes a crucial factor in the placebo effect, affecting the individual's ability for self-healing and accelerating the desired outcome (Humphrey 2002, 2; see further Kaptchuk 2002, 817; Gracely et al. 1985; Shapiro 1969; Kaptchuk and Eisenberg 1998; Crow et al. 1999; Di Blasi et al. 2001; Panagiotidou 2016a). In particular, in the Asclepius sanctuaries, specific preparatory steps, purifications and rituals were followed, which is likely to have enhanced patients' expectations, altered their psychological states, and prepared them for an 'extraordinary' divine experience.

Mental and Bodily Purification: Staying and Wandering in the *Asclepieia*

The supplicants who visited the Asclepius temples[26] in order to sleep in the *abaton*, would be exhausted by their journey and engrossed in their illnesses. Although the inscriptions mainly offer information on healing experiences during incubation, supplicants would probably stay in the sanctuary for some days before they entered the *abaton* (Horstmanshoff 2004b, 279; Nutton 2005, 110; Cilliers and Retief 2013, 81). During that time, they possibly ambled around in the sanctuary, talking with other people, observing the rituals performed by others, hearing healing stories, reading the inscriptions, and waiting for their own turn. There were also some mandatory preparatory rituals that they should perform in order to purify both their souls and bodies (Panagiotidou 2011, 130, 2021a; Von Ehrenheim 2015, 36–43; Renberg 2017, 249–258).[27] The god's demand for mental and bodily purification is underlined by Porphyry, where he describes the sacrifices in Epidaurus:

> It is necessary, therefore, that, being purified in our manners, we should make oblations, offering to the Gods those sacrifices which are pleasing to them, and not such as are attended with great expense. Now, however, if a man's body is not pure and invested with a splendid garment, he does not

---

26. Mainly those who travelled long distances from their homelands to the great *asclepieia*.
27. According to Patton (2004, 202), 'Intentional preparation and orientation were mandatory in ancient dream incubation'; see also Israelowich 2012, 151–152; Cilliers and Retief 2013, 75–76. On the Asclepius' demand for bodily purity and moral integrity, see Chamoux 2003, 335.

think it is qualified for the sanctity of sacrifice. But when he has rendered his body splendid, together with his garment, though his soul at the same time is not, purified from vice, yet he betakes himself to sacrifice, and thinks that it is a thing of no consequence; as if divinity did not especially rejoice in that which is most divine in our nature, when it is in a pure condition, as being allied to his essence. In Epidaurus, therefore, there was the following inscription on the doors of the temple:

Into an odorous temple, he who goes
Should pure and holy be; but to be wise
In what to sanctity pertains, is to be pure.

(Porph. *Abst.* II, 19, trans. Taylor 1823)

As Porphyry's quote indicates, the supplicants should undergo an initial purification before they offer sacrifices to the god. A bath at the holy spring was probably an appropriate means of purification, since water could release the soul from body dirt, and prepare it to communicate with the deity.[28] A fragmentary inscription from Pergamum implies that the supplicants should abstain from coitus for ten days, while there should be certain intervals of time between visits to the *asclepieion* and contacts with birth or death.[29] Furthermore, it was forbidden for women to give birth to their children within the borders of the holy precinct, and nobody was allowed to die within the *temenos*. These prohibitions reflect the general categories of purity and pollution in ancient Greek religious thought, according to which birth, death, coitus, menstruation, and certain foods

---

28. Cf. Pl. *Cra.* 405a-b: 'For in the first place, purification and purgations used in medicine and in soothsaying, and fumigations with medicinal and magic drugs, and the baths and sprinklings connected with that sort of thing all have the single function of making a man pure in body and soul' (trans. Fowler 1921); on the purificatory nature of ritual bathing at the Asclepius cult, see, for example, Dillon 1994, 245; Von Ehrenheim 2015, 36-40; Israelowich 2015, 117-118.

29. *IPerg.*, II, 264: 'let him enter into the Asclepius sanctuary ... he will have ten days [of abstinence from women ... days from child-givers ... days from funerals] ... entering, after bathing, if [he would like to find relief from his suffering] ... to be set free, let him purify completely' (trans. Edelstein and Edelstein 1998, T. 513); see Charitonidou 1973, 93; Dillon 1994, 244-245; Petsalis-Diomidis 2005, 204; Von Ehrenheim 2015, 25-36; Renberg 2017, 625-627. Similar restrictions were determined in two inscriptions found in Balagrae in Cyrenaica (*SEG* 20.759, dated to the second or third-fourth century AD; see Sokolowski 1973) and Thuburbo Maius in Africa (*ILAfr.* 225, dated to the second century AD; see Kleijwegt 1994, 210-211; Renberg 2017, 243-244, n. 326).

were conceived as pollutant in ritual contexts.[30] Supplicants, abstaining from all profane thoughts and behaviours, purified their souls and bodies, and washed away every kind of dirtiness through baths in the holy springs of Asclepius (see Ginouvès 1962, 352–357; Dillon 1994, 245; Von Ehrenheim 2015, 23–43; Renberg 2017, 239–249; Panagiotidou 2021a). Libations were also performed as a means of purification.[31] Then, the patients submitted their offerings which, as we have seen, might include poor, non-bloody dedications or lavish bloody sacrifices[32] in honour of Asclepius and the other gods who had an altar in his sanctuary (see Von Ehrenheim 2015, 49–73). An inscription describes the appropriate way in which the initial offerings should be made in Athens: 'Gods. The initial offerings are to be made in the following way: to Maleas three sacrificial cakes, to Apollo three cakes, to Hermes three cakes, to Iaso three cakes, to Aceso three cakes, to Panacea three cakes, to the dogs three cakes, to the huntsmen three cakes' (*IG* II(2), 4962, trans. Edelstein and Edelstein 1998, T. 515).

After the supplicants had offered sacrifices, they should take a second bath in order to be entirely purified.[33] When they had completed all the preparatory rites, they were dressed in white chitons, taking off their seal-rings and belts, being barefoot, holding laurels and bearing fillets on their heads (see Von Ehrenheim 2015, 75–78). Then they were bodily and mentally ready to enter the *abaton* and come into communication with the divine physician.[34]

---

30. On the categories of purity and pollution in ancient Greek religion, see, for example, Parker 1983; Burkert 1985, 77–79; Bendlin 2007, 178–189; Petrovic and Petrovic 2016. For the rules of purity before incubation, see Von Ehrenheim 2015, 25–35; Renberg 2017, 625–627.
31. Aristid. *Or.* L, 6: 'Thereupon purifications took place near the river by means of libations' (trans. Edelstein and Edelstein 1998, T. 518); on libations, see Parker 1985, 70–73; Von Ehrenheim 2015, 62–64.
32. For an example of the lavish bloody sacrifices, see Philostr. *V A* I, 10 = T. 517; see also Dillon 1994, 244, 146–247; Edelstein and Edelstein 1998, v. II, 190.
33. Paus. *Descr. Graec.* V, 13, 3: 'The same rule applies to those who sacrifice to Telephus at Pergamum on the river Caicus; these too may not go up to the temple of Asclepius before they have bathed' (trans. Jones and Ormerod 1918).
34. *IPerg.*, II, 264: 'to be free, let him purify completely ... in a white chiton and with brimstone, and with laurel ... with fillets which let him purify completely ... let him go toward the god ... into the great incubation room, the incubant ... with pure white sacrificial victims garlanded with olive shoots ... neither seal-ring nor belt nor ... barefoot' (trans. Edelstein and Edelstein 1998, v. I, T. 513); see further Dillon 1994, 245–246; Petsalis-Diomidis 2005, 205; cf. Mills 1984.

Reward Expectation: Assigning Salience to Random Events

In the wider context of the Asclepius cult, purificatory rituals and sacrifices were presented as important stages that paved the ground for the divine revelation and should precede the contact between supplicants and the divine healer during incubation. As indicated by Clifford Geertz's (1990, 91, 93) definition of religion, 'religious rituals' constitute 'culturally invented symbolic displays' which convey tangible 'conceptions of the world and imbue them with emotional and motivational significance' (cited by Deeley 2004, 245). Participation in the preparatory rituals that took place in the specific natural settings and architectural environment of the cult along with the impact of the anatomical votive offerings and inscriptions on the patient's expectations for healing and belief in Asclepius, the prospect of personal communication with the god during incubation as well as the subjective experiences of diseases, the fear of long-term suffering or death and the hope of salvation probably entailed high emotional arousal during patients' stay in the sanctuary (Panagiotidou 2021a).

According to the cognitive neo-association model,[35] emotional arousal can alter the ways in which various cognitive units – like perceptions, image-schemas, concepts, symbolic meanings, mental representations, episodic memories – are associated with each other, building up conceptual and cultural knowledge as well as experience of the perceptible world (Deeley 2004, 259). The dopamine arousal system seems to play a crucial role in this process, converting 'the neural representation of an external stimulus from a neutral and cold bit of information into an attractive or aversive entity' (Kapur 2003, 14). In particular, Shitij Kapur (2003), offering an account of psychosis, formulated the 'motivational salience hypothesis' of the dopamine system. According to this hypothesis, dopaminergic activity in the mesolimbic dopamine system of the brain mediates the 'attribution of salience' to external events and internal thoughts, attracting attention and affecting human behaviour toward a goal through its connection with reward or retribution (Kapur 2003, 14). In particular, increased dopamine secretion makes human perceptions of internal situations or external events seem extremely significant and meaningful, increasing the perceptual actuality of the relevant experiences (Kapur

---

35. On the cognitive neo-associationist approach to conceptualization and cultural learning, see, for example, Strauss and Quinn 1997.

2003, 14; Deeley 2004, 260). Kapur argues that an excessive release of dopamine takes place in the organisms of patients who suffer from psychosis, that is not caused or induced by current contexts, and leads to the attribution of aberrant 'salience and motivational significance to external stimuli' and internal representations and memories (Kapur 2003, 14).[36]

Quinton Deeley (2004, 260), expanding on Kapur's hypothesis in ritual settings, argues that especially during religious rituals, dopamine release depends upon and is in tune with the general social, cultural and symbolic contexts. Offering a modern insight on Clifford Geertz's (1990) definition of religion, Deeley suggests that rituals involve multiple sensory stimuli, and reinforce 'attention, arousal, and emotion' as well as 'semantic evocation and memory formation' (Deeley 2004, 257). Particularly, in religious rituals, a 'sensory route' is followed, and induces thinking and experience, 'orchestrating multiple reinforcing social-emotional signals and other stimuli'. Parallel to the sensory route, a 'semantic route' uses 'verbal and non-verbal symbols', which activate processing in the analogical right hemisphere in order to make sense of everything that happens and seems real but poorly understood (Deleey 2004, 263). Both of these routes mediate multiple cognitive and emotional processes, and particularly activate the mesolimbic dopamine system (Deleey 2004, 263) which makes the 'moods and motivations' induced during rituals seem particularly real (cf. Geertz 1990, 91, 93). Through this multiple affective and cognitive processing, the mesolimbic dopamine system is activated, allowing the assignment of salience to specific symbols, actions, objects and narratives, that seem particularly real and significant – perhaps more real and significant than ordinary reality (Deeley 2004, 260–262). As Deeley (2004, 245) puts it, these social, cognitive and neural processes mediate the transformation of religious ideas into beliefs.

In this light, healing events and symbolic meanings reported in the inscriptions from the *asclepieia* could indicate *similar* reactions and experiences likely resulting from increased dopamine secretion in the organisms of Asclepius' supplicants, who would have tended to interpret random events as particularly significant and meaningful facts.

An inscription from the Asclepius sanctuary at Epidaurus reports the case of a man from Kios who suffered from gout: '(A man) from Kios, gout.

---

36. On extreme dopamine release before and during psychotic episodes experienced by schizophrenic patients, see Strange 1992; Abi-Dargham et al. 2000; Greenfield 2000; Howard 2006.

This man, while he was awake, was walking over to a goose, which bit him in the feet and by making them bleed, made him well' (*IG* IV(2), 1, 122, XLIII, trans. LiDonnici 1995, B23).

This narrative conveys the story of a person who came to the *asclepieion*, suffering from the symptoms of a chronic illness, probably full of hopes and expectations of relief.[37] While he was in the sanctuary, he experienced an accidental event. However, such an event occurring in the wider healing, ritual context of the Asclepius temple, was perceived as a meaningful and significant experience by the patient, indicating divine intervention. The animal was perceived as guided by the god's will to cure his supplicant. This 'intensification of the sense of significance and meaningfulness' (Deeley 2004, 260) of a random experience would be mediated by activation of the mesolimbic dopamine system which facilitates the attribution of salience to events, attracting attention, guiding behaviour towards a goal, and being associated with reward. The patients probably hoped and expected divine help, and would have been prompt to trace signs of intentional communication and divine interventions in seemingly accidental occurrences,[38] and, further, to interpret random events as rewards for their belief in Asclepius' healing power.

This ascription of salience to seemingly random events is also implied in other stories from Asclepius' great temple at Epidaurus. 'Nicanor, lame. When he was sitting down, being awake, some boy grabbed his crutch and ran away. Getting up he ran after him and from this he became well' (*IG* IV(2), 1, 121, XVI; trans. LiDonnici 1995, A16). 'A mute girl. This girl, walking into the sanctuary, saw a snake moving away from one of the trees of the grove. She was filled with fear, and right away she yelled for her mother and father, …and left…' (*IG* IV(2), 1, 123, XLIV, trans. LiDonnici 1995, C1). 'Lyson of Hermione, a blind boy. The boy, while awake, had his eyes treated by one of the dogs about the sanctuary, and went away well'. (*IG* IV(2), 1, 121, XX, trans. LiDonnici 1995, A20). 'A dog cured a boy from Aigina. He had a growth on his neck. When he had come to the god, a dog

---

37. We should keep in mind that the story of the man from Kios – as well as other stories reported on the inscriptions – is not taken as a real event that actually happened at the Epidaurian *asclepieion*. Such healing narratives can be seen as records of potential instances of similar experiences that supplicants could have at the *asclepieia*.

38. As emphasized in the second chapter, tracing divine will for intentional communication with humans in seemingly random experiences comprises a fundamental element of the anthropomorphic perception of gods; see also Panagiotidou 2016b, 13–14.

from the sanctuary took care of him with its tongue while he was awake, and made him well' (*IG* IV(2), 1, 122, XXVI, trans. LiDonnici 1995, B6).

Particularly in the last three cases, the salience ascribed to the dogs and serpent would have been enforced by the human ability for symbolic thought (Deeley 2004, 246–250). Dogs and serpents were considered to be Asclepius' holy animals and symbols of his healing power (Kerényi 1959, 52–56; Meier 1967, 19–21). Executive abilities and processes, including 'attention, working memory, representation of context, temporal sequencing, abstraction, planning, and monitoring' (Deeley 2004, 247) – all involved in symbolic cognition – enabled Asclepius' supplicants to 'construct abstract or "higher order" conditional associations' (Deeley 2004, 247). In these associations, the signs of dogs, serpents or other animals and objects acquired special meanings as parts of a wider symbolic system which determined the connections between the signs (Deeley 2004, 247). Thus, patients would perceive dogs and serpents not just as ordinary animals idly wandering around, but as symbolic demonstrations of the god's willingness to help them by sending his own servants. And the god was eager to offer aid as a reward for the belief, behaviour, and actions of his supplicants.

Such impulsive attributions of salience to mental representations of stimuli associated with specific rewards, are mediated by dopamine, providing the motivational significance of rewards (Berridge and Robinson 1998, 309). According to Berridge and Robinson's (1998, 311, 313) hypothesis, 'dopamine projections from the substantia nigra and ventral tegmentum to forebrain structures such as the nucleus accumbens and neostriatum', re-determine the 'neural representations of conditioned stimuli' which are perceived as significant and meaningful events and motivate humans to pursue reward. In particular, neural systems, which are associated with dopamine and generate desire, 'interact with hedonic and associative learning components' generating the more complex 'process of reward' (Berridge and Robinson 1998, 313) (Figure 5).

In this view, dopamine projections in the brains of Asclepius' supplicants could attribute incentive salience to otherwise random events. Patients arriving at the *asclepieia*, expected to be cured from their sufferings and diseases. Activation of the dopamine mesolimbic and neostriatum systems would enforce their desire for relief and generate reward expectations assigning incentive salience to stimuli which could seemingly guide them to salvation. Appearances of animals, casual meetings with other people, or any kind of accidental events could be interpreted

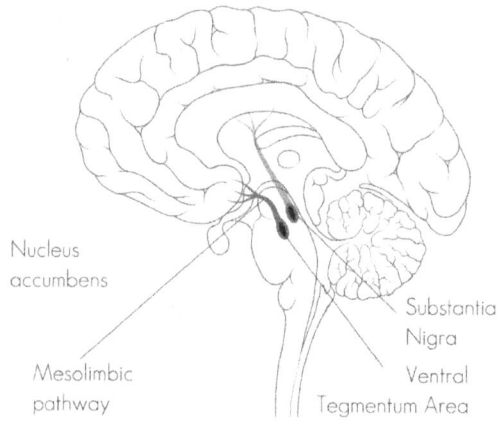

Figure 5 Mesolimbic dopamine system.

Source: edited by Nikos Katsikaridis

as significant, meaningful and purposeful through processes of reward learning and the ability of anticipating reward situations through associative correlations.[39]

However, dopamine projections and reward expectations with accompanying incentive salience attributions to stimuli would most likely reach their culmination in the incubation ritual, during which patients expected to meet Asclepius in person.

Conditioning, Intuitive and Cultural Expectations: The Healing Narratives

The inscriptions from the *asclepieia* conveyed healing narratives[40] about patients who supposedly had visited the sanctuaries in the past as well as to the illnesses, diseases and disabilities from which they suffered, and to their treatments by Asclepius (Paus. *Descr. Graec.* II, 27, 03).

---

39. Neutral triggers and random events are invested with significance and unique meanings in a wide range of high emotionally arousing rituals. See, for example, Xygalatas' research (2012) on the signs (σημάδια) reported by the participants in the ritual of Anasthenaria in Agia Eleni, a village in Northern Greece.

40. On the significance of the healing narratives in Asclepian medicine, see, for example, LiDonnici 1992, 25–41; Dillon 1994; Martzavou 2012, 177–204.

The best-preserved collection of *iamata* comes from the Epidaurian *asclepieion* and was inscribed on three free-standing steles in the second half of the fourth century BCE.[41] According to Lynn LiDonnici (1995, 65–69), these narratives were collected and recorded in groups possibly by the priests, but they reflect different sources for their content and formations (see also Martzavou 2012, 177–178; Renberg 2017, 172). As LiDonnici notes, certain groups of inscriptions sharing common themes, but differing in linguistic terms, probably constituted the written forms of oral tales which circulated among the god's devotees, temple authorities, and other people who lived or worked around the sanctuary. Supplicants probably heard stories about the healing powers of Asclepius and their manifestation in certain individual cures, and spontaneously transmitted these tales, enhancing patients' expectations of healing. The priests and cult servants would have also been interested in communicating these stories in their attempt to convince the supplicants of the effectiveness of their visits to the sanctuary (Dillon 1994, 240; LiDonnici 1995, 50–60, especially 52). Some of the cases of healing recorded by the latter were possibly based on relevant pictorial representations on the votive offerings, following the pattern of the oral stories. Among the Epidaurian *iamata*, there are also groups of narratives which resemble each other linguistically, but differ in themes. As LiDonnici suggests, these inscriptions might be originally produced by professional artisans and merchants who worked around the sanctuary. The supplicants could order their inscriptions to the votive makers and sellers who used stereotypic stories, customizing them by the addition of the name and specific case of the buyer (Figure 6).[42]

Among the earliest Epidaurian *iamata*, there are some records of peculiar human conditions which Asclepius healed in miraculous ways.[43] There is, for instance, the following story:

---

41. Pausanias (*Descr. Graec.* II, 27, 03) reported that he saw six such steles during his visit to the Epidaurian sanctuary and he mentioned that there should be more such collections in the past; see Herzog 1931, 2; Habicht 1969, 155; Siefert 1980, 326; Longrigg 1993, 20–21; Dillon 1994, 240. Healing inscriptions have been also found at the *asclepieia* of Lebena (*ICr* I, xvii, 8–24), Pergamum (*IPerg.*) and Rome (*IGUR* 148).
42. On the origins of narratives and possible explanations of their groupings, see LiDonnici 1995, 60–65, 74–75.
43. In two inscriptions, for example, the god appears to help two women, who were pregnant for years, to give birth to their children after they went as supplicants to his sanctuary (*IG* IV(2), 1, 121, I, II). On rational explanations of 'protracted pregnancies', see Demand 1994, 93–94.

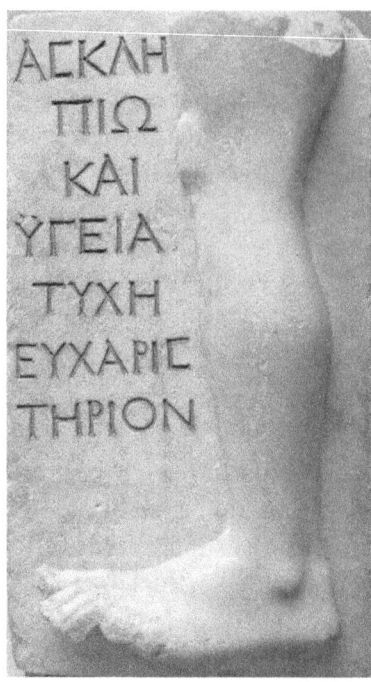

Figure 6 Votive relief with an inscription dedicated to Asclepius and Hygeia. Found in 1828 in same sanctuary in Milos.

Source: British Museum, public domain, via Wikimedia Commons

> [A man] came as a supplicant to the god who was so blind in one eye that, while he still had the eyelids of that eye, there was nothing within them and they were completely empty. Some of the people in the sanctuary were laughing at his simple-mindedness in thinking that he could be made to see, having absolutely nothing, not even the beginnings of an eye, but only the socket. Then in his sleep, a vision appeared to him. It seemed that the god boiled some drug, and then drew apart his eyelids and poured it in. When day came he departed with both eyes.
>
> (*IG* IV(2), 1, 121, IX, trans. LiDonnici 1995, A9)

This narrative is highly revealing regarding both people's expectations and the cures performed at the *asclepieion*. Reporting other supplicants' reactions to a patient's hope of healing, the story assumes the common intuitive expectations of the biological and physiological construction and function of the human body that would have been shared by people in Graeco-Roman antiquity. Humans constantly act as naive physicists (see, for example, Hayes 1979) and psychologists (see, for example, Churchland

1979, 1981, 1984; Stich 1983), sharing intuitive understandings of natural laws and others' behaviours, emotions and motives in order to make sense of both natural and social surroundings. Thus, we can imagine that the supplicants laughed at the blind man's silly hope of a cure, because they intuitively expected that nothing can be created *ex nihilo*, and consequently it was inconceivable for an eye to grow in an empty eye-socket. However, in the inscription, Asclepius was presented to disprove their intuitive expectations and attract their attention – as well the attention of later visitors who would read the inscription.[44] He appeared to use a vague but ordinary medical means – pouring some drug in the patient's eyesocket – and by this to perform a treatment that violated the natural laws that govern the world (Panagiotidou 2016b, 17–18).

The story of Ambrosia, referred in chapter 3, also reports her predisposition to the prospect of cure: 'Ambrosia..., blind of one eye... she ridiculed some of the cures as being unlikely and impossible, the lame and the blind becoming well from only seeing a dream. Sleeping here, she saw a vision. It seemed to her the god ... cut her sick eye and poured a medicine over it. When day came she left well' (*IG* IV(2), 1, 121, IV trans. LiDonnici 1995, A4).

In this narrative, the supplicant herself appears to laugh and challenge the possibility of healing. However, contrary to the previous story, now the reason of dispute was not the cure that seemed inconceivable, but the employed healing method that did not seem to be the appropriate – 'merely seeing a dream'. Ambrosia's reaction would have derived from the cultural expectations about the medical practices that can lead to cure – expectations she would have acquired through cultural learning and conditioning with human medicine.[45] Dreams were used as useful diagnostic tools by many Hippocratic doctors, but they were not considered to have significant therapeutic value (e.g. *Regim.* IV; Oberhelman 1987, 2013, 25–26; Holowchak 2001; Hemingway 2008, 134–135; Harris 2009, 243–244, 284; Petridou 2014). Therefore, for those who were familiar with human medicine, the use of dreams by Asclepius appeared to be an extraordinary means of healing that would violate their cultural expectations about the

---

44. Cf. Boyer's theory on counterintuitive concepts, which I mainly examined in the second chapter.
45. Once again, I need to note that I do not approach this particular narrative as an actual event, but as a record that reflects potential reactions of some of the Asclepian supplicants.

therapeutic methods and practices employed by professional doctors and would thus grab their attention.[46]

Familiarity is largely achieved through conditioning, a mode of learning during which a neutral stimulus is unconsciously paired with a potent stimulus through repetition.[47] Repeated consultations with doctors may be paired with the employment of specific treatments that are accompanied by symptoms relief and cure (Crow et al. 1999, 3). Despite a probable exaggeration,[48] most of the inscriptions represent Asclepius as applying medical techniques and remedies to patients' inflicted bodily parts and carrying out specific surgical procedures commonly employed by human doctors. The *iamata* record simple (e.g. *IG* IV(2), 1, 122, XL) to more complex cases (e.g. *IG* IV(2), 1, 121, XIII). Asclepius appears to pour drugs into his supplicants' eyes (*IG* IV(2), 1, 121, IV, IX, XVIII, 122, XL), to operate on patients cutting open their belly (*IG* IV(2), 1, 122, XXIII, XXV, XXVII) or breast (*IG* IV(2), 1, 121, XIII), removing and re-attaching their bodily parts (*IG* IV(2), 1, 122, XXIII, XXXII), taking materials off their bodies (*IG* IV(2), 1, 121, XII, 122, XXV, XXX, XXXII) and draining their bodily fluids (*IG* IV(2), 1, 122, XXI) (Panagiotidou 2016c). Although in many of the recorded cases Asclepius appears to use his superhuman powers and to perform superhuman treatments, the reference to his medical procedures that resemble those of doctors could have induced conditioned symptom relief

---

46. Although dreams were a common means of healing employed by gods and heroes in their sanctuaries, they were not usually employed by doctors as therapeutic tools. Asclepius was considered to be the supreme doctor who employed the means, practices and methods used by his human counterparts. For people who were conditioned in human medicine and expected that Asclepius would behave as a doctor, healing dreams would have violated those people's expectations. About the effects that the violations of cultural expectations have on attention and memory systems see the research of Porubanova-Norquist and her colleagues (2013, 2014) mentioned in the second chapter; see also Panagiotidou 2016b, 17–18.

47. On conditioning, see, for example, Rescorla 1988; Voudouris, Peck and Coleman 1990; Ader 1997; Montgomery and Kirsch 1997; Brody and Brody 2000; Siegel 2002; Klinger et al. 2007; Porro 2009, 2–3.

48. As noted, in some cases, Asclepius appears to employ ordinary medical means to extremely difficult conditions that would have been – or actually were – rejected by doctors. Or he seems to heal illnesses and ailments that his human counterparts had failed to cure (e.g. *Anth. Pal.* VI, 330 = T. 404; Ael. *Fr.* 89 = T. 399; see Wickkiser 2008, 58–61; Renberg 2017, 23–24).

and thereby placebo responses in the supplicants who participated in the ritual of incubation.[49]

Healing narratives have also been fragmentarily preserved at the *asclepieion* in Lebena which had certain affiliations with Epidaurus.[50] The tales were inscribed onto the walls of the *stoa* and are dated in the second century BCE. The texts were probably collected by the priesthood from individual votive offerings on wood, and display certain linguistic and thematic similarities with the inscriptions from Epidaurus. They mainly differ from the Epidaurian *iamata* in the ways in which the cures were performed by Asclepius. In particular, the god appears to administer certain plants to his patients, while, at least in one case, he uses cupping instruments (LiDonnici 1995, 47–48). This shift from the use of unknown drugs in Epidaurus to certain pharmaceutical plants in Lebena may reflect the influence of Hippocratic medicine to the Asclepius cult (Israelowich 2015, 59) as well as the progress in pharmacology and pharmacopoeia from the Hellenistic period (see Scarborough 1991; Horstmanshoff 2004b; Cilliers and Retief 2013, 78; Renberg 2017, 226-238).[51] Furthermore, conditioning with mundane medicine along with the increase of the Asclepius' reputation as a divine physician would have transformed people's expectations about the treatments offered at his sanctuaries.[52]

Furthermore, both the Epidaurian *iamata* and the healing inscriptions from Lebena mention certain diseases and disabilities which Asclepius

---

49. In the second chapter, we briefly saw how the refusal of treatment by human doctors could have led to negative conditioning in usual medical practices; on negative conditioning, see Crow et al. 1999, 3 referring to Wickramasekera 1980; Turkkan and Brady 1985.

50. Approximately 22 narratives are preserved. Originally, there should be many more inscriptions on the walls of the *stoa*; see LiDonnici 1995, 47–48.

51. According to Renberg (2017, 214-218), there is evidence that Asclepius was thought to perform miraculous interventions even during the Hellenistc and Roman periods. The phenomenal alterations of his healing methods may be attributed to the different kinds of sources that are preserved from different places and eras. In any case, it seems that Asclepius operated both as healing deity and divine physician and did not abandon any of these qualities with the passage of time.

52. This difference between the Epidaurian *iamata* and the inscriptions from Lebena might also reflect local preferences and traditions in these cities; the *asclepieion* in Epidaurus attracted visitors from almost every part of the Greek world, and addressed people coming from various conceptual origins and traditions, while Lebena was visited by supplicants coming from a narrower geographic area (LiDonnici 1995, 47–48). In addition, people of different social ranks, economic status and education may have had different levels of familiarization and conditioning with professional doctors; see Renberg 2017, 228-229.

could cure. These cases mostly refer to chronic ailments,[53] including pregnancy problems and sterility, eye diseases, muteness and deafness, paralyses and lameness, ulcers, tumours, pus and festering sores, gout, stones in the penis, stomach disorders, worms in the belly, leeches in the chest, dropsy and epilepsy, chronic headaches, insomnia, even lice and baldness (*IG* IV(2), 1, 121–123; *ICr*). The chronic nature of the representations of these illnesses indicates that many patients would have been suffering for a long time before they asked the aid of Asclepius (e.g. *ICr* I, XVII, 17 = T. 439; Wickkiser 2008, 59; Renberg 2017, 213–214; Panagiotidou 2021b). Their despair would have led them to the *asclepieia* in order to seek relief from a doctor whose healing powers were considered to be much greater than those of human physicians.

Along with the alterations of healing methods employed by Asclepius, the very nature of the cures he performed also appears to gradually change. Henk S. Versnel (2011, 406–407) has aptly pointed out an internal difference among stories of *supernatural* healings that appeared to break natural laws and violate human intuitive understandings of the world, and stories of *superhuman* cures that seemed to surpass the healing abilities of human doctors and mundane medicine. The Epidaurian *iamata* demonstrate such a transition from more supernatural to more superhuman treatments, a shift that is manifested in the healing inscriptions from Lebena in which Asclepius appears to employ or prescribe precise medical procedures and remedies.[54] This alteration might further reflect an increased conditioning of the people of Graeco-Roman antiquity with human medicine and the development of specific cultural expectations about doctors.[55]

---

53. On Asclepius' specialization on chronic ailments, see Edelstein and Edelstein 1998, V. II, 169; Schäfer 2000, 264–265; Nutton 2005, 109; Wickkiser 2008, 58–61; Cilliers and Retief 2013, 74; Renberg 2017, 213–214; Panagiotidou 2021b; cf. Cael. Aurel. *Morb. Chron.* Praef. 2 = T. 364. Gerald Hart (2000, 8) and Edward Tick (2001) suggest that many of these ailments might have psychosomatic origins; see also Oberhelman 2013, 74, 85–86.
54. The alteration of Asclepius' healing practices is also reflected in Aelius Aristides *Orationes* that describe treatments performed at the Pergamene *asclepieion* in the second century AD. Contrary to the immediate cures reported in the Epidaurian *iamata*, in the *Orationes*, Asclepius appears mostly to prescribe treatments and to give advice and prescriptions to his supplicants (see Horstmanshoff 2004a). The gradual reduction of miraculous healings that is manifested in the Hellenistic *iamata*, culminated in the healing narratives of Graeco-Roman period which report cures that are attributed to Asclepius but largely depended on self-administered remedies; Cotter 1999, 23, citing Kee 1983, 89.
55. On the public performances of doctors and people's access to medical procedures, see, for example, Cilliers and Retief 2013, 77–78.

At the same time, the patients who had visited *asclepieia* would have communicated their experiences and the healing narratives heard from others or read in the inscriptions to their friends and members of their social networks, thus contributing to the development and spread of common cultural expectations about Asclepius. Thus, through social interaction and cultural learning, the newcomers would have already formed an idea of Asclepius and expected from him to behave as a doctor and to also use the means and techniques of mundane medicine (Lloyd 1979, 40–41; Israelowich 2015, 60).[56]

Conformity Bias and Normative Cognition: Reading the Inscriptions

In the context of the Asclepius cult, the healing inscriptions were presented as fragments of personal narratives of people who visited the *asclepieia* and were cured by Asclepius in the past. We can trace in these stories' implicit evidence about supplicants' health problems, desires, hopes, expectations, and rewards. However, although the healing inscriptions might have been originally individual dedications to the sanctuaries, as mentioned above, they were collected by the priests and cult authorities and inscribed together as public documents of Asclepius' healing power. In this way, the inscriptions comprised a valuable means of propaganda that was intended to manipulate supplicants' conformity bias and expectancies, attempting to convince them that their health recovery was feasible even in the most incredible cases, if they behaved in the appropriate way and believed in Asclepius.[57]

That patients should be convinced of the potentiality of recovery was suggested in some stories of the inscriptions, which refer to cases of supplicants who came to the *asclepieia* and were suspicious about the power of Asclepius to heal them:

> A man who was paralyzed in all his fingers except one came as a supplicant to the god. When he was looking at the plaques in the sanctuary, he didn't believe in the cures and was somewhat disparaging of the inscriptions.

---

56. That Asclepius used the techniques of mundane medicine is also indicated by votive offerings found in Pergamum and Rome; LiDonnici 1995, 48.
57. On the 'didactic nature' of the *iamata*, see Dillon 1994; cf. Błaśkiewicz 2014; Molen 2019.

> Sleeping here, he saw a vision. It seemed he was playing the knucklebones below the temple, and as he was about to throw them, the god appeared, sprang on his hand and stretched out the fingers. When the god moved off, the man seemed to bend his hand and stretch out his fingers one by one. When he had straightened them all, the god asked him if he would still not believe the inscriptions on the plaques around the sanctuary and he answered no. 'Therefore, since you doubted them before, though they were not unbelievable, from now on', he said, 'your name shall be 'Unbeliever'. When day came he left well.
>
> (*IG* IV(2), 1, 121, III, trans. LiDonnici 1995, A3)

Narratives like this possibly were intended to convince patients who suffered from chronic diseases and disabilities, and might have been despaired of the possibility of salvation, to believe in the healing power of Asclepius (cf. Dillon 1994, 257; Błaśkiewicz 2014, 35-36; Renberg 2017, 213-214). The divine physician could cure even the most unbelievable cases and was so benevolent that he offered aid even to disbelievers (Wells 1998, 37). However, the disparagement and mockery of his treatments was an inappropriate behaviour which was punished by the god (cf. *IG* II(2), 1, 121, IV).

The healing inscriptions included also stories in which the supplicants did not have a coherent dream sent by the god (see Martzavou 2012, 183, 188). Instead, they experienced divine healing in unexpected ways during their every-day life. Sostrata from Pherai (*IG* IV(2), 1, 122, XXV = T. 423, XXV), for example, slept in the *abaton*, but she had no clear dream. Later, after she left the sanctuary, she underwent a healing experience on her way back home. Such stories conveyed by the inscriptions probably were intended to comfort the supplicants who could not have the desired healing dream or vision from the god (Martzavou 2012, 188-189). Furthermore, they attempted to dissuade incubants' disappointment and loss of their belief in Asclepius which would have hurt the god's reputation.

At the same time, the healing narratives presented the supplicants as being responsible for not being cured by the god. If the patients had not received a healing dream from Asclepius, this was because they had not sufficiently purified their bodies and minds before incubation. Or perhaps their requests had not been clearly determined (*IG* IV(2), 1, 121, II, Panagiotidou 2016c).

Furthermore, the internalization of particular beliefs about the *abaton* was further promoted in some stories from the Epidaurian *iamata*. The *abaton* was the place in the temple where the ritual of incubation took place. It was inaccessible to visitors. Only incubants had the permission to enter. The narratives conveyed in the inscriptions, indicated the possible consequences if someone disobeyed this rule: 'Aischines, when the suppliants were already sleeping, went up a tree and peered over into Abaton. Then he fell out of the tree and impaled his eyes on some fencing …'[58] (*IG* IV(2), 1, 121, XI, trans. LiDonnici 1995, A11).

Stories like this indicate the intention of the Asclepius cult to affect the *reflective* and *normative cognition*[59] of supplicants in order to discourage them from entering the *abaton* without permission,[60] and the modulation of supplicants' conformity bias and reflective beliefs might further have impact on their bodily responses.[61]

Priming Before Incubation: Primes in the Healing Narratives

In any case, the healing inscriptions displayed at the *asclepieia* attempted to encourage, inspire hope and convince patients of the effectiveness of Asclepian therapy.[62] In addition, since the healing narratives were not spontaneous expressions of the individuals who had experienced incubation, but were organized and recorded by the cult officials (Martzavou 2012, 182, 185), they were articulated in such a way in order to communicate a complex sequence of precepts and ideas that linked health recovery to specific scripts of actions and outcomes. In this way, the healing

---

58. Compare the secrecy around the Eleusinian mysteries and the case of a man who found death when, moved by curiosity, climbed up a rock trying to look over the walls of Eleusis, during celebrations; Ael. *Frag.* 58, 8; Dillon 1994, 248.
59. On normative cognition, see the Introduction; cf. Jensen 2010, 2013, 2016.
60. On the way in which religious norms are primed and embodied, and affect the believers' attitudes and behaviour, see Shariff and Norenzayan 2007; McKay et al. 2010.
61. Modern research in brain imaging, which investigates the neurobiology of social constructivism and its impacts on the human brain and body, reveals the ways in which collective rules and constraints affect the states and reactions in the human body (Jensen 2010, 328, 2013, 2016; Panagiotidou 2014b, 20; further Zahn et al. 2009).
62. On the inscriptions as a means of arousing the emotions of hope and confidence to Asclepius' supplicants, see Martzavou 2012, 177–204. Dillon (1994, 257) has also emphasized that the *iamata* were intended to encourage 'those pilgrims who were very ill to believe that there was some hope of their recovery'; cf. Błaśkiewicz 2014; Molen 2019.

narratives could be viewed as means of priming the new supplicants for their potential subsequent experiences in the *abaton* (Panagiotidou 2021a).

Priming is defined as 'a nonconscious form of memory that involves a change in a person's ability to identify, produce or classify an item' (material object, abstract notion, concept or experience) 'as a result of a previous encounter with that item or a related item' (Schacter, Dobbins and Schnyer 2004, 853). Priming increases the 'speed of response' to semantically associated primes (Storbeck and Clore 2008, 2; see further Neely 1990; Klauer and Musch 2003). In particular, priming briefly activates a representation which becomes accessible to the person who has no awareness of the prime or how he or she is being affected by it (Randolph-Seng and Nielsen 2009, 240). Priming effects entail implicit perception and representation of a stimulus (visual, auditory, olfactory, etc.), subliminal retention in memory of the particular features of this perceived stimulus,[63] establishment of associations between two or more stimuli presented in the same conditions, and later deployment of certain responses which accompanied previous encounters with the same stimuli (Schacter, Dobbins and Schnyer 2004, 853).

Various ordinary stimuli, like odours, sounds, objects, words or even patterns of behaviours and activities – like rituals – can prime humans, thus leading them to share common subjective experiences (Raafat, Chater and Frith 2009, 425). In social and therefore religious contexts, 'subtle primes' implicitly influence participants 'in an assimilative manner' (Randolph-Seng and Nielsen 2009, 240), and can generate similar experiences and exegetical reasoning.[64]

The supplicants, arriving at the *asclepieia* with an intrinsic religious orientation, expected to receive divine healing. As long as they prepared themselves for the ritual of incubation, they would have been occupied by feelings of impatience and anxiety, triggered by the prospect of entering the sacred space of the *abaton* where their encounter with the god was about to happen.[65] The healing narratives, written in the inscriptions

---

63. Priming generates associations in semantic memory which are automatically activated in both semantic and affective priming (Neely 1990; Bargh 1997; Storbeck and Clore 2008, 2).
64. Modern research has shown that priming of religious concepts reduces cheating (Ariely 2008; Bering, McLeod and Shackelford 2005; Randolph-Seng and Nielsen 2007), while it can promote trust and altruism (Shariff and Norenzayan 2007; Ruffle and Sosis 2010).
65. On the *abaton* as a place 'not to be trodden', and the potential 'emotional tension' caused by the feelings of 'fear of transgressing a limit', 'awe' by entering a sacred space and 'anticipation and hope for a cure', see Martzavou 2012, 180.

and orally circulating among visitors, patients and the temple *sacristans* conveyed the main information about supplicants' appropriate behaviour as well as Asclepius' interventions, therapeutic methods and possible health outcomes. Beyond the obvious accounts, healing narratives subliminally operated as effective means of priming the experiences that the supplicants would expect to have in the *abaton*. Most inscriptions had embedded certain words[66] which referred to a stage of sleep (ἐγκαθεύδω, ἐγκατακοιμάομαι) during which Asclepius appeared to perform his treatments in 'dreams' or 'visions' (ἐνύπνιον, ὄψιν) (Panagiotidou 2021a). In addition, the inscriptions implied the association between Asclepius and human medicine by extensively using the medical terminology that was widely used by Hippocratic doctors.[67] These words primed particular images, actions, emotions and mental states which could be stored as long-term conceptual representations in supplicants' semantic memory. These representations could be recalled when the supplicants would be in a context similar with that described in the inscriptions (cf. Schacter, Dobbins and Schnyer 2004, 854). Entering the *abaton*, incubants could structure their personal experiences according to what they had previously heard or read about others' encounters with Asclepius (Panagiotidou 2013, 2021a; cf. Randolph-Seng and Nielsen 2009, 241).

Body Fragmentation: Anatomical Votive Offerings and Localization

Beyond the narrative inscriptions, the Asclepius sanctuaries were full of other kinds of votive offerings dedicated by the supplicants who wished to express their gratitude to the god. Thank-offerings varied from bandages, stones, dice, vessels, figurines, clay cocks, silver pigs and cups to reliefs, statues and even buildings.[68] These offerings were displayed as the material evidence of their dedicators' visits and cures – or cure requests – at the *asclepieia* (LiDonnici 1995, 41; Dignas 2007, 169).

---

66. On the language, words and similar forms of the inscriptions, see Wells 1998, 31–39, 79–85, 100–102.
67. On the words used in the inscriptions and a possible chronological grouping, see LiDonnici 1995, 76–82; on the common medical vocabulary used in mundane and temple medicine, see Israelowich 2015, 52–53.
68. On the votive offerings that filled up the ancient Greek sanctuaries, see Van Straten 1981.

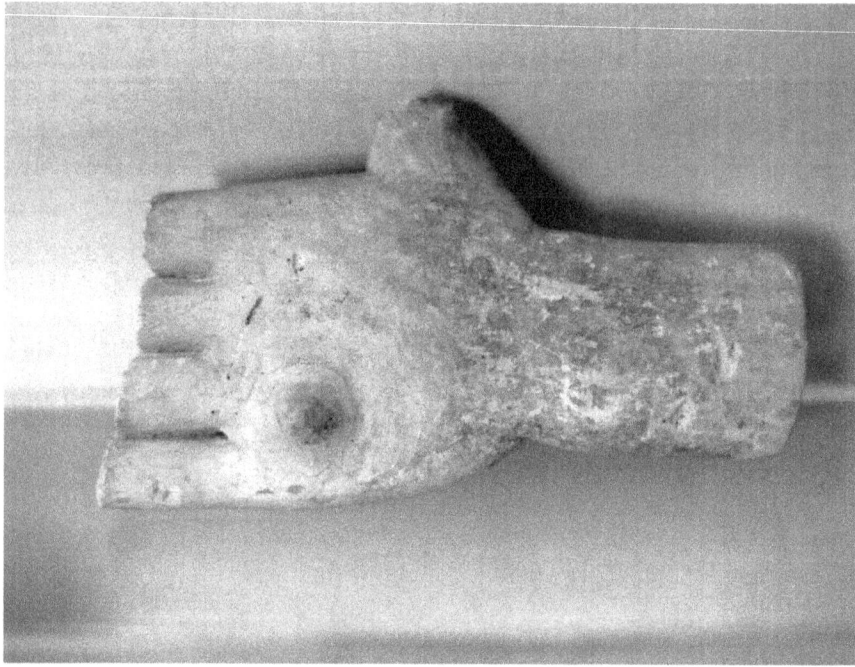

Figure 7 Votive terracotta to Asclepius, fourth century BCE. Archaeological Museum of Ancient Corinth.

Source: Zde, CC BY-SA 4.0, https://creativecommons.org/licenses/by-sa/4.0, via Wikimedia Commons

Among the dedications, hundreds of anatomical votive offerings[69] have been revealed in many of the Asclepius temples, representing almost every part of the human body (Figure 7).[70] Their shapes, materials and sizes varied. The most usual patterns included representations of bodily parts on stone relief tablets, carved metal plates or even three-dimensional clay

---

69. People who had been cured by Asclepius could dedicate a material representation of their healed body parts as thank-offering to the god. However, as Aelius Aristides (*Or.* VI, 38, pp. 66–67) reports, patients could dedicate a replica of their suffering body part in asking to be cured by the god (see Van Straten 1981, 103, 105; Schörner 2015, 406).

70. The greatest amount of anatomical votive offerings has been found at the *asclepieia* in Corinth and Athens. On the anatomical ex votos at the Athenian *asclepieion*, see Van Straten 1981, 108–113; Aleshire 1989, 33, 40. The offerings unearthed in Corinth are unique, since they are three-dimensional, life-size, made from terracotta (see Van Straten 1981, appendix, A 15.1–118). However, similar dedications were possibly made at the great sanctuaries of Asclepius in Epidaurus, Pergamum, and on Kos (Hughes 2008, 219).

or stone effigies. These offerings were designed to hang on the walls of the temples and *stoas*, and other places within the sanctuary, and even on the trees and small steles constructed for this reason (Rynearson 2003, 7; Schörner 2015, 406, 409; Panagiotidou 2021a).

Viewing these offerings would impress the supplicants who arrived at the sanctuaries. The representations of the inflicted body parts as fragments implied the localization of illness or disease to specific parts of the patients' bodies (Rynearson 2003, 7-8; Schörner 2015, 406, 407-408). This sense of body fragmentation indicated a perception of health and disease (Rynearson 2003, 7-8) in the cult context, and could possibly mediate the enhancement of placebo effects. According to Humphrey's (2002, 2005) approach, placebos tend to be effective, when they are applied to specific parts of the human body (Humphrey 2005, 2; see Chapter 1). Thus, the representations of the inflicted body parts would imply the focus of the Asclepius medicine, not on the general structure and processes of the human organism, but on its specific fragments that suffered from particular diseases, illnesses or disabilities. This localization of the disease and treatment stood in contrast to the current precepts and methods used by Hippocratic doctors, who attempted to restore health through regimen of the whole body instead of remedies applied to specific parts, in which the symptoms might be localized (Rynearson 2003, 4-5, 8; Wickkiser 2008, 47; Schörner 2015, 406, 407-408). Thus, looking at the fragmentary votive offerings, the supplicants were indirectly suggested to focus on their body parts that were infected by illness. It was implied that the disease or illness had not inflicted their whole bodies. Their disabilities were localized only on specific body parts, and recovery was possible through divine intervention.

Furthermore, the anatomical votive offerings would not just be perceived as representing parts of the patients' bodies that had been healed by Asclepius. They could also be conceived as pictorial fragments of the life-narratives of people who, suffering from the symptoms of their illnesses, had visited the *asclepieia* and found salvation (Rynearson 2003, 8; Schörner 2015, 406; Panagiotidou 2021a). In this view, each anatomical votive would be perceived as the trace of the presence of its dedicator at the sanctuary, and the proof of his or her healing by Asclepius. The supplicants could dedicate their offerings after they had been cured by the divine physician, and their dedication would have been their last action in the sanctuary before they returned to their ordinary life (Rynearson 2003, 9). Thus, the presence of the represented body part would have further signified the absence of a whole body belonging to a living person who had been restored to health by Asclepius. The patient, leaving the *asclepieion*, on the one hand, would dedicate an anatomical votive to the god in order to remain symbolically in the sanctuary as a substitute of his or her real body part in order to ensure the integrity of his or her whole body, when he or she would leave (Rynearson 2003, 9–10; Hughes 2008, 224). Aelius Aristides, clearly testifies this operation of votive offerings as substitutes of the living body in the sacred space of the *asclepieia*:

> And (he indicated) [Asclepius] that it was also imperative to cut off part of the body itself in behalf of the safety of the whole. This, however, would be too great a demand and from it he would exempt me. Instead, I should take off the ring which I was wearing and offer it to Telesphorus. For this would do the same as if I offered the finger itself. Furthermore, I should inscribe on the band of the ring "Son of Cronus". After this there would be salvation ...
> (Aristid. *Or.* XL VIII, trans. Edelstein and Edelstein 1998, T. 504)

The perception of these anatomical votive offerings by the newcomers, on the other hand, was the witness of the presence of other people at the *asclepieia* and the cure of the latter's diseases by Asclepius. In short, the anatomical votive offerings were intended to advertise the feasibility of cure, since they were presented as being offered by people who had suffered from similar illnesses and were healed by Asclepius in the past.

The sense of body fragmentation was also implicitly evident in many inscriptions reporting healing cases in which Asclepius applied remedies and treatments to specific organs and parts of patients' bodies. In this way, both inscriptions and anatomical votive offerings not only proclaimed Asclepius' superhuman healing power. They further operated as a means of priming and indirect suggestion of specific precepts, concepts and expectations in the supplicants (Panagiotidou 2021a). They induced mental representations, implicit memories and relative expectations about what was possible for them to experience during incubation. In this view, hearing the healing narratives, viewing the votive offerings, and discussing both of them played a crucial role in the preparation of supplicants for the ritual of incubation.

Chapter 5

The Culmination of Incubation

Creating the Miracle

Beginning with the affliction from a disease, the experience of the symptoms of an illness and suffering from sickness (see Chapter 1), mediated by cultural influences and social interactions outlining potential routes to recovery (Chapters 2 and 3), and reaching the decision to visit an *asclepieion* where the supplicant received multiple sensory stimuli and social influences (Chapter 4), led finally to the ritual of incubation. Incubation was the culminating event of the patients' stay in the *asclepieia* during which the divine physician was supposed to perform his treatments. Not all the supplicants would have slept in the *abaton*. Some of them, however, would have undergone the ritual of incubation hoping to receive a healing dream or vision.

In this final chapter, I examine how all the cultural influences, social interactions and patterns of thought that mediated patients' decisions to resort to the *asclepieia*, and the particular elements of the Asclepius cult context, would have affected patients' cognition forming the experience of incubation within the *abaton*. The ancient sources do not provide a clear image of the ritual nor explicit evidence about what happened in the *abaton*. However, I suggest that taking into account the findings of neurocognitive research on the impacts of the realm of wakefulness on the dreaming brain may enable us to fill in the gaps in our historical knowledge and articulate reasonable assumptions about how the supplicants might have experienced their stay in the *abaton*. In particular, perception of Asclepius as a benevolent superhuman doctor and the patients' expectations in attracting his interest and receiving a cure could have played a crucial role in the inducement of placebo responses (*placebo drama*). Such responses could have been activated in the sensory deprived environment of the *abaton* where the suggestive images, stories, thoughts, and expectations could have formed experiences that could have been perceived as extraordinary or even miraculous in an altered state of consciousness. Once again, I do not claim that the suggested scenarios actually took place in the *abaton*, but I intend to outline how patients' perceptions, thoughts, knowledge, information and expectations could have framed their personal needs, thus making them more amenable to placebo effects or just most suggestible to believe that Asclepius could help them.

Incubation: Entering the *Abaton* and the Healing Experience

Upon the nightfall, supplicants entered the *abaton* in order to sleep there and wait for a healing dream or vision from Asclepius (Figure 8). Records and descriptions of patients' healing experiences in the *abaton* are preserved from the fifth century BCE to the end of Graeco-Roman antiquity. Although these testimonies were probably enriched by the authors' poetic

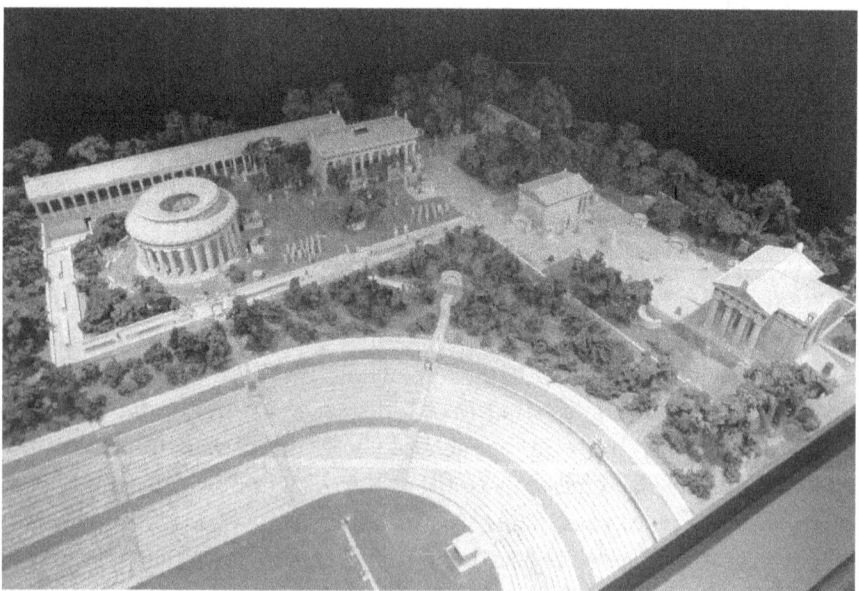

Figure 8 Model of the *asclepieion* at Epidaurus, Greece, 1936.

Source: Science Museum A632959, CC BY 4.0, https://creativecommons.org/licenses/by/4.0, via Wikimedia Commons

phantasy or the zeal of the cult devotees, they outline a rough impression of incubation (see Edelstein and Edelstein 1998, v. II, 145–158; Cilliers and Retief 2013, 76; Renberg 2017, 238–239; Steger 2018, 91–102).

Among the literary sources, Aristophanes' *Plutus* offers the most detailed description of the ritual. Plutus, the protagonist of the comedy, visited the *asclepieion* of Aigina, hoping to be cured from blindness. His servant, Carion, reports to his master's wife his experiences at the sanctuary. Despite the comical nuance of the narrative and the sarcastic attitude of the author mainly towards the god's priests, Carion sketches out the general form of incubation (Ar. *Plut.* 633–747 = T. 421; see Edelstein and Edelstein 1998, v. II, 151; Martzavou 2012, 177; Cilliers and Retief 2013, 79, 87).

Soon after Plutus arrived near the temple, feeling miserable, he was brought by his servants to the sea, and took a bath in the cold water. Afterwards, the company went to the precinct, and offered honey-cakes and bakemeats on the altar. Then they entered the *abaton*, and laid down on rough beds. Many other patients, suffering from every kind of sickness, were also there, waiting to be healed. Soon after, a servant of the temple put out the lights, and bade everyone fall asleep and remain recumbent and silent, whatever noise might be heard. Then Asclepius entered the *abaton* followed by his assistants and two snakes (see Ar. *Plut.* 653–657 = T. 421).

In broad terms, Aristophanes' description can be considered to be the pattern of incubation that took place in the Asclepius temples.[1] This pattern is partially confirmed by the *iamata* (see further Horstmanshoff 2004a, 326–331; Martzavou 2012, 177). The supplicants entered the *abaton* and stayed alone, isolated from the external world. In the lights of candles, they lay down on pallets, full of excitement and expectations for their oncoming communication with the deity. And when the lights were blown out, they remained in the dark and silent *abaton* expecting Asclepius to approach them in a dream or vision (Edelstein and Edelstein 1998, v. II, 149–158; Panagiotidou 2011, 130–131, 2021a, 2021b; Cilliers and Retief 2013, 76; Von Ehrenheim 2015, 94–96; Renberg 2017, 258).

---

1. Aristophanes' description is reminiscent of the Classical relief from the *asclepieion* of Piraeus; see Mitropoulou 1977, 63–64, No. 126, and fig. 183. *LIMC* II, 'Asklepios', No. 105; on the ritual of incubation in the Epidaurian and Pergamene *asclepieia*, see also Cilliers and Retief 2013, 76–77.

Most testimonies report that the divine physician appeared in his supplicants' sleep in human-like semblance (see Holowchak 2002, 158; Renberg 2010, 36–37; Cilliers and Retief 2013, 78; Panagiotidou 2016b, 13, 2021b; cf. *IG* IV(2), 1, 12; Aristid. *Or*. IV 50). Resembling the appearance of his statues, most times he was imagined as a mature bearded man[2] who approached incubants holding his staff, while sometimes he was accompanied by his sacred serpents. He addressed the patients with his harmonious voice (Suidas, *Lexicon*, s.v. Δομνῖνος), having a gentle, calm expression on his face. Such an image of the god is described by Ovid, who narrates the invocation of Asclepius by the Roman embassy sent to Epidaurus:

> as dusk dispelled the lingering light, and darkness covered the countries of the earth with shadow, then, in your dreams, Aesculapius, god of healing, seemed to stand before your bed, Roman, just as he is seen in his temple, holding a rustic staff in his left hand, and stroking his long beard with his right, and with a calm voice, speaking these words: 'Have no fear! I will come, and I will leave a statue of myself behind. Take a good look at this snake, that winds, in knots, round my staff, and keep it in your sight continually, until you know it! I will change into this, but greater in size, seeming as great as a celestial body should be when it changes ...'
> (Ov. *Met*. XV, 651–662, trans. Kline 2014)

In other cases, Asclepius appeared in his supplicants' dreams as a handsome young man who saved them from suffering (*IG* IV(2), 1, 121, XVII = T. 423, XVII, *IG* IV(2), 1, 122, XXV = T. 423, XXV). He approached the incubants with good intentions, he engaged in discussions (cf. Oribasius, *Coll. Med*. 45, 30, 11–14) and sometimes teased and laughed with them having a humorous mood (*IG* IV(2), 1, 121, VIII = T. 423, VIII). In many inscriptions, mainly in the earliest ones, Asclepius is represented as immediately operating on and healing the patients[3] (e.g. *IG* IV(2), 1, 121, XVIII, XII = T. 423, XVIII, XII; cf. Panagiotidou 2011, 131).

He quite often intervened in person in the healing process. Sometimes he touched his patients with his divine hand, or kissed their ailing bodily parts (*IG* IV(2), 1, 122, XXXI, XLI = T. 423, XXXI, XLI; cf. Cilliers and Retief 2013, 80; Renberg 2017, 218–220). In other cases, the treatments were

---

2. As noted in the second chapter, this was the typical iconic representation of human doctors throughout Graeco-Roman antiquity; cf Cilliers and Retief 2013, 78.
3. The potentiality of actual surgical operations recorded in the *iamata* has been examined by Helen Askitopoulou and her colleagues (2002); see also Cilliers and Retief 2013, 79–80.

performed by Asclepius' sacred animals – dogs who licked the patients' suffering body parts or snakes who penetrated into their bodies (*IG* IV(2), 1, 121, XIV = T. 423, XIV; Panagiotidou 2011, 131, 2016b, 13).[4]

Sometimes, however, the incubants received puzzling dreams and needed to consult the priests or *sacristans* in order to decipher the divine will and treatment (see Von Ehrenheim 2015, 99–101). As noted in the previous chapter, especially in the Hellenistic and Roman times, Asclepius increasingly appeared in dreams or visions to prescribe specific remedies that the supplicants should use after incubation. This change of the Asclepian medical practices in the Graeco-Roman era is indicated by a well-preserved inscription dated in the second century CE. The inscription describes the complex prescriptions that Asclepius ordained to Marcus Julius Apellas, a sick resident of Asia Minor, who suffered from dyspepsia, in order to restore him to health (Wells 1998, 38–39):

> When I arrived at the temple, he told me for two days to keep my head covered…; to eat cheese and bread, celery with lettuce, to wash myself without help, to practice running, to take lemonpeels, to soak them in water, near the (spot of the) *akoai* in the bath to press against the wall, to take a walk in the upper portico, to take some passive exercise, to sprinkle myself with sand, to walk around barefoot, in the bathroom, before plunging into the hot water, to pour wine over myself, to bathe without help and to give an Attic *drachma* to the bath attendant, in common to offer sacrifice to Asclepius, Epione and the Eleusinian goddesses, to take milk with honey. When one day I had drunk milk alone he said, 'Put honey in the milk so that it can get through'. When I asked of the god to relieve me more quickly, I thought I walked out of the *abaton* near (the spot of) *akoai* being anointed all over with mustard and salt, while a small boy was leading me holding a smoking censer, and the priest said: 'You are cured but you must pay up the thank-offerings'. And I did what I had seen, and when I anointed myself with the salts and the moistened mustard, I felt pains, but when I bathed, I had no pain. That happened within nine days after I had come. He touched my right hand and also my breast … To gargle with a cold gargle for the uvula – since about that too I had consulted the god – and the same also for the tonsils. He bade me also inscribe this. Full of gratitude, I departed well.
>
> (*IG* IV(2), 1, 126, trans. Edelstein and Edelstein 1998, T. 432)

---

4. On Asclepius' epiphanies in the form of his sacred animals, see Petridou 2014, 294–295; cf. Cilliers and Retief 2013, 80–81.

Asclepius often appeared to use salves and drugs which he kept in his medical chest.[5] His prescriptions included either ordinary remedies or drugs invented by him.[6] He could employ natural substances, like water, as well as drugs, used by human doctors, on his patients during their dreams, but the effects of these remedies might be extraordinary. In general, his prescriptions varied significantly depending on the ailments they intended to cure. His treatments sometimes differed from the suggestions of his mortal disciples, opposed somehow paradoxically to human theory and empirical knowledge (see Edelstein and Edelstein 1998, v.II, 153–154; Cilliers and Retief 2013, 80; Panagiotidou 2021b). Aelius Aristides consulted a doctor about the prescriptions which he had received from Asclepius in a dream or vision, since he found them peculiar:

> Having seen these things, when morning dawned, I call the physician Theodotus; and as he comes, I described to him my dreams. He was astonished at how strange they were, and he was at a loss to what to make of them, since it was wintertime and, too, he was anxious over the great weakness of my body; for I had already been confined to my home for many months. For this reason, it seemed to us to be good idea to summon the *sacristan* Asklepiacus also.
> (Aristid. *Or.* XLVIII, 31–35, trans. Edelstein and Edelstein 1998, T. 417)

The appearance of Asclepius, described in the inscriptions and literary sources, was not threatening. His kind attitude towards his supplicants, and his eagerness to provide aid even to those who doubted or disputed[7] his healing powers would enhance the patients' trust to the divine physician, and their conviction that a cure could happen through their personal communication with him in the *abaton*.[8]

---

5. Ar. *Plut.* 708–711: 'Asclepius did the round of the patients and examined them all with great attention; then a slave placed beside him a stone mortar, a pestle and a little box' (trans. O'Neill 1938; see Edelstein and Edelstein 1998, v. II, 153).
6. Aelius Aristides, for instance, attributed to the god the discovery of a well which could cure various diseases (*Or.* XXXIX, 14–15 = T. 409).
7. Cf. *IG* IV(2), 1, 121, IV, IX = T. 423, IV, IX.
8. On Asclepius' epiphanies, see Cilliers and Retief 2013, 78; Petridou 2014, 292–296.

Asclepius and His Supplicants: An Empathic Doctor–Patient Relationship

The ways in which the inscriptions describe Asclepius and the personal healing experiences of his supplicants during incubation reveal the latter's feelings towards the former. These feelings would further modulate the expectations of the newcomer patients of their coming encounter with the divine physician during incubation. Beyond the treatments and drugs employed or prescribed for the various illnesses, the personal relationship between the divine doctor and his patients could have had an immediate therapeutic effect (Di Blasi et al. 2001, 757). Hippocrates outlined this potentiality of the doctor–patient encounter: 'For some patients, though conscious that their condition is perilous, recover their health simply through their contentment with the goodness of the physician' (*Praec*. VI, trans. Jones 1868).

Although modern clinical research is mainly interested in evaluation of the surgical and pharmacological interventions, neglecting the potential effects of doctor's attitudes towards a patient's condition, there is evidence that the interaction between doctors and patients can significantly affect the latter's health outcomes (Turner et al. 1994, 1609–1614; Di Blasi et al. 2001, 757).

Howard Leventhal and his colleagues (1982, 55–86) presented a theoretical model of self-regulation, and the mechanisms for the appraisal of symptoms as a way of understanding the effects of the healthcare interactions (see Panagiotidou 2021b). According to them, when individuals experience the symptoms of an illness, they are possessed by feelings of anxiety and uncertainty, while they try to make sense of what happens to them, of the possible causes and duration of the symptoms, and of the potentiality of their treatment. Then, they usually consult the doctors, who can practise both cognitive and emotional care in parallel with the employment of medical means. Cognitive care refers to the means used by physicians to influence patients' perception of their illness and their expectations of the effects of the treatment. These expectations can be positive, negative, or even neutral depending on the doctor's comments about the effectuality and safety of the treatment.[9] Emotional care refers

---

9. For instance, if doctors would describe a treatment as 'good, safe and effective', patients would have positive expectations about its outcome. On the other hand, however, if doctors would describe the treatment as 'dangerous, unsafe and ineffective' with 'potential

to the mode of consultation adopted by the healthcare givers in order to reduce the negative emotions of fear and anxiety felt by patients. 'Support, empathy, reassurance, and warmth' in doctors' behaviour help patients to feel safe, and encourage the elimination of negative emotions (Di Blasi et al. 2001, 758; see further Leventhal, Nerenz and Strauss 1982, 55–86). The interactive operation of cognitive and emotional care can amplify the effectiveness of a treatment prompting the human organism to activate its own self-healing systems (Di Blasi et al. 2001, 760; cf. Panagiotidou 2021b).

Kaptchuk (2002) has identified five essential components that influence the effectiveness of both active medical interventions and placebos: patient, healer, relationship between patient and healer, nature of the ailment, treatment and settings in which the treatment is performed. These factors comprise the *placebo drama* which could have amplified effects in certain conditions (Kaptchuk 2002, 817–818), like those prevailing in the Asclepius cult.[10]

The patient is the 'protagonist' in each healing case (Kaptchuk 2002, 818). Modern research indicates that patients' expectations can affect both active and inactive (placebo) interventions. These expectations are grounded in the person's pre-established beliefs formulated in the context of the treatment, and his or her own previous experiences as well as the experiences of his or her acquaintances, friends and relatives (Crow et al. 1999, 4). Particularly, alternative medical practices, contrary to conventional medicine, promote an exaggerated perception of the possibility of healing which draws out the patient's anticipation about the health outcome without being constrained 'by the laws of normative physics' (Kaptchuk 2002, 818). In this view, Asclepius' supplicants were called upon to believe in the healing power of the benevolent divine physician, not because this power was confirmed by logical argumentation and objective criteria, but because they were eager to be 'taken into the imagination and lived with, if only for a time' (Kaptchuk 2002, 818, citing Kirmayer 1993, 161–195).

Furthermore, they were asked to adhere to the treatments offered by the god in order to find relief from their illnesses. Patients should participate

---

side effects', patients would have negative expectations of its employment (Di Blasi et al. 2001, 758). If doctors would avoid characterizing a treatment and offer neutral information about it, patients would have neutral expectations about its outcome (Di Blasi et al. 2001, 758; see further Leventhal, Nerenz and Strauss 1982, 55–86).

10. For an application of the theory of the placebo drama to the Asclepius cult, see Panagiotidou 2021b.

in the healing process by following the divine prescriptions. This was the part that they should play in the *placebo drama*, and its accomplishment was a matter of personal responsibility.[11] This sense of responsibility could promote the adherence to the god's instructions, and activate the placebo response. In particular, the patients who suffered from chronic illnesses and had a negative experience with mundane medicine for a long time (Rescorla 1988; Voudouris, Peck and Coleman 1990; Ader 1997; Montgomery and Kirsch 1997; Klinger et al. 2007; Porro 2009, 2-3), found reason to hope for recovery by visiting the Asclepius sanctuaries which provided 'an opportunity for "deconditioning" from the previous unsuccessful medical experiences' (Kaptchuk 2002, 818) through personal communication with the god (see Panagiotidou 2016b, 16-17).

Positive expectations, adherence to a prescribed regimen, and the sense of personal responsibility constitute, as Kaptchuk suggests, the patient's personal contributions to the placebo effect (Kaptchuk 2002, 817-818; see further Czajkowski and Chesney 1990; Horwitz and Horwitz 1993; Gallagher, Viscoli and Horwitz 1993; McPherson, Britton and Wennberg 1997; Mattocks and Horwitz 2000) (Figure 9).

The practitioner, for his part, should present him or herself as heroic healer in order to facilitate the patient's placebo response (Kaptchuk 2002, 818; see further Shapiro 1969, 215-248). Although further research is required, recent studies indicate that the doctor's attitude towards a particular illness and the employed treatment, can significantly affect health outcomes.[12] Especially the healers of alternative medical practices are often more enthusiastic and optimistic than conventional doctors (Kaptchuk 2002, 819). Asclepius seems to follow this pattern. He was presented as the omnipotent divine physician, who employed the most advanced medical methods and healed even diseases that his mortal counterparts could not. His appearance in the dreams or visions of his supplicants enhanced his perception as a saviour god who provided aid to anyone seeking salvation. He did not hesitate to apply even the most extreme treatments, and he was sure about their success, if patients adhered to his instructions and accomplished their commitments. The idea that the god could heal

---

11. On the significance of patient's adherence to the applied treatments, see Czajkowski and Chesney 1990; Horwitz and Horwitz 1993; Gallagher, Viscoli and Horwitz 1993; McPherson, Britton and Wennberg 1997; Mattocks and Horwitz 2000; Kaptchuk 2002, 818; cf. Renberg 2017, 24-25.

12. On the relevant RCTs, reviews and studies, see Kaptchuk 2002, 818-819.

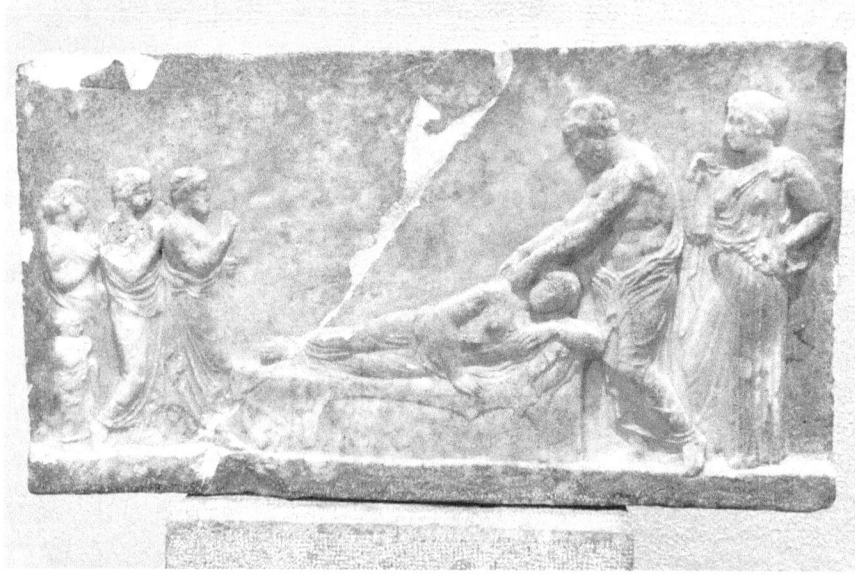

Figure 9 Votive relief of Asclepius healing a patient. *Asclepieion* of Piraeus, ~350 BCE.

Source: George E. Koronaios, CC BY-SA 4.0, https://creativecommons.org/licenses/by-sa/4.0, via Wikimedia Commons

any kind of illness or other disability and that the potential failure of a treatment derived from patients' deficiencies is obvious in the following inscription:

> A three-year pregnancy. Ithmonika of Pellene came to the sanctuary for a family. Sleeping here she saw a vision. It seemed that she asked the god if she could conceive a daughter, and Asclepius answered that she would and that if she asked anything else that he would do that as well, but she answered that she didn't need anything more. She became pregnant and bore the child in her stomach for three years, until she came again to the god as a supplicant, concerning the birth. Sleeping here she saw a vision. The god appeared, asking whether everything she had asked had not happened and she was pregnant. She had not asked anything about the birth, and he had asked her to say whether there was anything more she needed and he would do it. By since now she had come to him as a supplicant for this, he said he would do it for her. Right after this, she rushed out of the *Abaton*, and as soon as she was outside the sacred area, gave birth to a daughter.
>
> (*IG* IV(2), 1, 121, II, trans. LiDonnici 1995, A2)

In this narrative, Asclepius appears to be a benevolent god who was both able and eager to fulfil any request of his supplicant. If he did not do that in the first place, it was because the supplicant was not precise in her demand. The appearance of Asclepius as a healer with good intentions, ready to accomplish every petition, probably reassured his supplicants that their salvation was possible, if they knew exactly what to ask for.[13]

According to Kaptchuk, when both the healer and the patient perceive each other's beliefs and actions as reliable, the placebo drama can be more effective. The doctor–patient encounter is underlined in many studies as an influential factor in health outcomes.[14] The common expectations and attitudes towards the health problem being shared by the doctor and the patient during discussions as well as the former's explicit diagnosis and assurance that recovery is possible, would accelerate the process of recovery or the feeling of relief (Kaptchuk 2002, 819; see further Bass et al. 1986, 43–47; Finkler and Correa 1996, 199–207).

The nature of illnesses which were cured by Asclepius probably could benefit from placebo effects. Modern researchers conclude that the presence of subjective symptoms with no recognizable physical causes, chronic diseases, and emotional disorders are curable by placebo responses. Particularly, chronic pain, headache, gout, insomnia, chronic digestive problems, and other illnesses, which are mentioned in the *iamata*,[15] are among the ailments which are considered to be amenable to placebo effects. Even persons with common illnesses like cold, strains, and twists, can experience a faster recovery responding to the treatment, and thus they perceive the enhanced effectiveness of the offered treatment (Kaptchuk 2002, 820).

---

13. On this inscription and the emotions which would arise to the readers, see Martzavou 2012, 184–185.
14. On the doctor-patient interaction and its importance in placebo effect, see, for example, Kaplan, Greenfield and Ware 1989, 110–127; Stewart 1995, 1423–1433; Ong et al. 1995, 903–918.
15. Once again, it is necessary to emphasize that the healing narratives reported in the inscriptions are not taken as real cases that were treated by Asclepius, but as sources that provide evidence about the kinds of illnesses and diseases that the divine physician was represented as being able to cure. The reported stories include extraordinary ailments that could not be cured by placebo effects or any other means of treatment, and the methods employed by Asclepius were not always feasible. But as noted many times, such stories were a means of propagation of Asclepius' superhuman powers and of manipulation patients' thoughts, memories and expectations.

Furthermore, the treatment and its settings can modulate the effects of placebo performances, since they influence the patient's beliefs about the received care. Elaborate actions, like surgeries, can generate placebo effects, offering a sense of the healer's drastic intervention. But also more ordinary processes like prescriptions can have similar responses, while the way in which a treatment is administered can influence 'its perceived action' (Crow et al. 1999, 4).

In the Asclepius cult, the sacred place of the *abaton* was covered by a veil of mystery, where the power of the god was revealed (cf. Patton 2004, 203–206). Each healing case had a certain 'intervention scenario' in which Asclepius provided an active treatment (cf. Kaptchuk 2002, 820). His treatments included hazardous surgical interventions as well as prescriptions which tended to be extremely complex, thus increasing the intensity of the placebo effect.

Although modern research in placebo effects is far from conclusive (Kaptchuk 2002, 820–821), it seems that the ritual of incubation, at the heart of the Asclepius cult, had potent performative efficacy which would generate enhanced placebo responses in its supplicants. For the patients who believed in the healing power of Asclepius, the Asclepian therapy might 'provide a superior placebo' (Kaptchuk 2002, 821) which would be actualized in their sleep.

Healing Dreams or Visions: Ancient Views and Modern Theories

Dreams were the most essential component of the ritual of incubation. When patients entered the *abaton*, they expected Asclepius to visit them in their sleep. In this condition, the incubants believed that the god would immediately perform his treatment or prescribe a certain regimen that they should follow upon awakening.[16]

The diagnostic value of dreams was also recognized by the Hippocratic doctors.[17] The author of the *Regimen* IV draws a distinction between the

---

16. For the dreams and visions that the Asclepius supplicants could have in the *abaton* and the cognitive mechanisms which could have mediated dreaming experiences, see Panagiotidou 2021a.
17. On the role of dreams as means of diagnosis and prognosis in the *Corpus Hippocraticum* (in *Regim.* IV as well as in other less known passages), see Hulskamp 2013; for a comparison between the use of dreams as prognostic tools in the Hippocratic texts and in the *iamata*

divine dreams which are sent by the gods, and the non-divine dreams, which are generated by alterations or disturbances of the internal balance of the body during everyday activities, expressed during sleep. In this view, the divine dreams are amenable to religious interpretations. Non-divine dreams, on the other hand, have bodily origins and are within the field of medical explanation. The author's remarks indicate the way in which Hippocratics conceived the state of sleep, and used dreams in their medical practice:

> He who has learnt aright about the signs that come in sleep will find that they have an important influence upon all things. For when the body is awake the soul is its servant, and is never her own mistress, but divides her attention among many things, assigning a part of it to each faculty of the body – to hearing, to sight, to touch, to walking, and to acts of the whole body; but the mind never enjoys independence. But when the body is at rest, the soul, being set in motion and awake, administers her own household, and of herself performs all the acts of the body. For the body when asleep has no perception; but the soul when awake has cognizance of all things – sees what is visible, hears what is audible, walks, touches, feels pain, ponders. In a word, all the functions of body and of soul are performed by the soul during sleep. Whoever, therefore, knows how to interpret these acts aright knows a great part of wisdom.
>
> Now such dreams as are divine, and foretell to cities or to private persons things evil or things good, have interpreters in those who possess the art of dealing with such things.
>
> Such dreams as repeat in the night a man's actions or thoughts in the daytime, representing them as occurring naturally, just as they were done or planned during the day in a normal act – these are good for a man. They signify health, because the soul abides by the purposes of the day, and is overpowered neither by surfeit nor by depletion nor by any attack from without. But when dreams are contrary to the acts of the day, and there occurs about them some struggle or triumph, a disturbance in the body is indicated, a violent struggle meaning a violent mischief, a feeble struggle a less serious mischief. As to whether the act should be averted or not, I do not decide, but I do advise treatment of the body. For a disturbance of the soul has been caused by a secretion arising from some surfeit that has occurred.
>
> (*Regim.* IV, lxxxvi–lxxxviii, trans. Jones 1923)

---

of Epidaurus as well as for the doctors' intention to establish their superiority in the interpretation of prognostic dreams, see Pearcy 2013.

Therefore, the Hippocratic doctors believed that the non-divine dreams were indicative of physical health and warned the dreamer about the onset or process of a disease. The physical symptoms influenced the dreaming imagery, and the doctors could diagnose a disease through the correct interpretation of the images and signs appearing in dreams (Holowchak 2002, 136; cf. Oberhelman 1987; Hulskamp 2013; Renberg 2017, 27–28).

Modern research seems to confirm some aspects of the Hippocratic theory of dreaming, as it is presented in *Regimen* IV. Although dreams can be reported as vivid experiences by dreamers (Nordin 2011, 231; see further Hartmann 1998), the bodily systems of attention, motion, and memory cease their functions during sleep (Krippner and Combs 2000). Motor output is constrained only to toes and fingers as well as to the eyes, whose rapid movement gave the name of the relevant phase of sleep in which the most vivid dreams are observed (REM sleep as opposed to non-REM sleep) [18] (Krippner and Combs 2000, 400). In addition, the brain actively suspends its sensitivity to exteroceptive stimulation (Flanagan 1997, 102; Krippner and Combs 2000, 400). Some neurophysiological evidence, however, indicates that acoustic stimuli are lightly perceived in REM sleep, an observation which could throw light into the processes through which external events are incorporated into the dreaming context (Flanagan 1997, 104).

According to Kahn, Krippner and Combs's (2000, 8) theory of the psychophysiological and cognitive structure of dreams, as long as the brain is isolated from external sensory inputs, patterns of activity can loosen in forms that are mostly based on the internal conditions of the body (Krippner and Combs 2000, 401–402; see further Antrobus 1990, 3–24). The dreaming brain rests on 'natural patterns of self-organized activity which often reflect the residual moods, stresses, and concerns of waking life' (Krippner and Combs 2000, 401). These patterns of activity are experienced as narratives unfolding during dreams (Combs and Krippner, 1998; Krippner and Combs 2000, 402). Krippner and Combs (2000, 402–403) suggest that dreaming narratives are composed of experiential components, like thoughts, perceptions, emotions, and memories, which interact and combine with each other during dreaming, thus generating new experiential components. And although the conditions under which they are

---

18. REM sleep is the rapid eye movement phase of sleep, as opposed to nREM sleep, in which movements of the eyes are not observed. For this distinction and the association of each state of sleep with dreaming, see Hobson and Stickgold 1994, 2; Krippner and Combs 2000.

activated differ from those in waking states, the dreaming and waking patterns of brain activity share the essential principles of their creation (Krippner and Combs 2000, 402).

In particular, during REM sleep, Hobson and his colleagues have observed that aminergic neurochemicals (serotonin and norepinepherine), which dominate in waking states and cause extensive inhibition in brain activity, are constrained (Hobson and Stickgold 1994, 1–2; Krippner and Combs 2000, 403). This decrease of aminergic modulation in the brain further facilitates the inhibition of working memory,[19] which allows rapid alterations in the dreaming plots. Working memory, along with other higher cognitive abilities, is localized in the prefrontal cortex, the activity of which shows a remarkable reduction in REM sleep (Krippner and Combs 2000, 403; see further Braun et al. 1998). While dreaming, individuals attend to the narrative without question or speculations about the future. They are not surprised by the bizarreness of what they experience, while their attention and self-reflection decrease (Krippner and Combs 2000, 404; on dream 'bizarreness' see Hobson and Stickgold 1994, 3).

Simultaneously, in a sleeping state, the cholinergic neurochemical acetylcholine makes the brain amenable to facile activation, allowing it to associate emotions, memories and fantastic elements together with higher ingenuity than in waking, free from the restrictions of everyday reality (Krippner and Combs 2000, 403; cf. Hobson 1994). In parallel, although the activity in the prefrontal cortex is reduced, parts of the limbic system, which is mainly associated with emotions, are particularly active (Krippner and Combs 2000, 404; see further Braun et al. 1998).

Furthermore, certain regions of the brain which mediate the generation and processing of visual images show increased activity during REM sleep. In particular, the adjacent (parastriate) regions, which are believed to play a fundamental role in 'the conscious experience of vision' (Krippner and Combs 2000, 405; see further Crick and Koch 1995; Revonsuo 1998), seem to be vigorously activated, while the primary visual cortex of the occipital lobe shows a significantly decreased activity in comparison to visual activity in waking (Krippner and Combs 2000, 404–405). According to Hobson and his colleagues, activity in the parastriate area also participates in dreaming imagery (Krippner and Combs 2000, 405; cf. Hobson, Pace-Schott and Stickgold 2000), while, as Braun and his colleagues

---

19. The decrease of aminergic modulation reaches 50% in nREM sleep and almost 100% in REM sleep (Krippner and Combs 2000, 404; see further Hobson 1988).

(1998) suggest, the anterior cingulate cortex and the right parietal lobe, which mediate the regulation of attention, are extensively activated in images during REM sleep (Krippner and Combs 2000, 404). In addition, ponto-geniculo-occipital waves (PGO waves), which are highly repressed in waking state and nREM sleep, send stimuli to the brain's visual system during REM sleep (Hobson and Stickgold 1994, 1) (Figure 10).

In this condition, the dreaming brain, cut off from daily external stimuli, is particularly susceptible to 'subtle influences' coming from the internal organism (Krippner and Combs 2000, 407). Residual memories and emotions, fleeting perceptions and primed experiences can be activated during sleep and connected to each other, forming the content of dreaming narratives (Krippner and Combs 2000, 401, 408). There is also evidence that slight biological influences can find expression in dreaming imagery, sending signals about the internal condition of the individual's organism (Krippner and Combs 2000, 408; see further Smith 1986).

Hobson and Stickgold (1994, 8) have defined dreams as sequences 'of sensations, images, emotions and thoughts passing through a sleeping person's mind'. Hallucinatory visual and auditory imagery and 'a sequence of perceptions' which resembles the form of a story or scenario are experienced by the dreamers during REM sleep (Hobson and Stickgold 1994, 8). However, the same mental activity does not take place during all the phases of sleep. Recent evidence indicates that humans dream also during

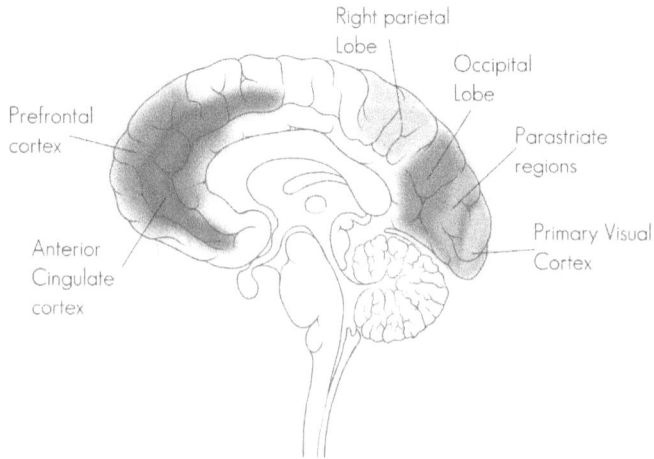

Figure 10 The dreaming brain.

Source: edited by Nikos Katsikaridis

nREM sleep, which resembles REM sleep to the extent that it can generate dreams, but its mental activity is more similar to the waking state (Krippner and Combs 2000, 405). Individuals, who wake up during nREM sleep, often report that they were not sleeping but thinking about something. However, the polysomnographic evidence suggests that these individuals were asleep, and therefore their mental ability could be described as 'nondreaming sleeping mentation' (Hobson and Stickgold 1994, 8).

Focusing on consciousness during dreaming, Cicogna and Bosinelly (2001, 33–34) suggest that dreams are generated by the interaction between three major processes: (1) the bottom-up activation of the elements of long-term memory and to a minor degree of the embedded external and internal stimuli, (2) which are interpreted through a top-down processing that re-activate the conceptual knowledge of the dreamer and generate new mnemonic contents, (3) which are further translated into images, words and emotions comprising the phenomenal experience and shaping the oneiric plot through effective control, selection and memory activity. The dreamer is aware of the phenomenal settings of the dream, namely of the objects and the events which comprise the oneiric plot as well as of his or her own presence in the scene and his or her thoughts and feelings about the other objects. Thus, the dreamer has also an awareness of his or her own self (self-awareness), since he or she participates in the action, and observes the unfolding events. However, the dreamer is not aware that these experiences are only the products of his or her own mental activity (meta-awareness).[20] Thus, the oneiric reality is illusory, since it draws information not from the actual external world, but from the internal milieu of the dreamer (Cicogna and Bosinelly 2001, 30). After waking up, individuals are able to recall the content of the oneiric episodes and to recognize their own cognitive conditions during dreaming, while they can also make 'post hoc distinctions on the qualities of waking and sleeping experiences' (Cicogna and Bosinelly 2001, 38).

Although modern research has not yet reached a full understanding of the neurobiology, physiology, cognition and mental activity of the dreaming brain, the above-mentioned descriptions offer valuable insights which could illuminate some aspects of the dreams that Asclepius' supplicants

---

20. With the exception of lucid dreams in which the dreamer is aware that he or she is dreaming (Cicogna and Bosinelly 2001, 26, 29).

would have at his sanctuaries.[21] Dreams during incubation were considered to be generated by the body and the physical condition of the sleepers and involved the appearance of the healing deity or his representatives who directly transmitted important information about the disease and its treatment. Allegorical images, which were interpreted by the oneirocritics or the mortal doctors,[22] were seldom included in incubants' dreams. However, the healing inscriptions, since they were not spontaneous records of the dreamers, do not offer grounds for a study of the dreams experienced by Asclepius' supplicants (Harris 2009, 107–108).

On the contrary, the oneiric diary written by Aelius Aristides includes oneiric reports which resemble the dreams that someone would expect to experience at the *asclepieia* in the second century CE. (Harris 2009, 120; Harrisson 2013, 47). His *Orationes*, composed around 150 CE, include the records of his frequent visits to healing sanctuaries in his attempt to recover his health.[23]

Andrew M. Holowchak has underlined the main features of the Aelius Aristides' oneiric tales, which indicate that these stories possibly have not been extensively revised, and would correspond to the real dreams that the orator experienced. According to Holowchak, many of Aristides' dreams are self-laudatory, and would reflect the accomplishment of a personal

---

21. A first, relatively brief, medical-neurocognitive account of Asclepius' supplicants' dreams was presented by Cilliers and Retief (2013, 82–85) that along with the cognitive mechanisms noted by Hobson and his colleagues takes into account Askitopoulou and her team's (2002, 7) claim that psychotropic-narcotic substances and drugs were used at the *asclepieia*.

22. For the interpreters of dreams during Graeco-Roman antiquity, see, for example, Renberg 2015.

23. Aelius Aristides' *Orationes* comprise a unique case of autobiographical diary which has attracted the interest of modern scholars and has elicited various approaches and interpretations of the work (see, for example, Phillips 1952, 23; Festugière 1954, 85–154; Dodds 1965, 41–45; Behr 1968; MacMullen 1976; Holowchak 2002, 156–157; Petsalis-Diomidis 2010; Israelowich 2012; Downie 2013a, 2013b; Tagliabue 2016; Petridou 2018) as well as of its author's personality (see, for example, Baumgart 1874; Michenaud and Dierkens 1972). Although the *Orationes* primarily comprise a literary work, which reflects the wider cultural and religious contexts in which it was produced, some scholars suggest that the oneiric descriptions may be seen as reports of the actual dreaming experiences of the author (see, for example, Holowchak 2002; Harris 2009, esp. 118–122; Stephens 2012). At this point, I employ Holowchak's (2002) approach and I make a few observations about that possibility. For a biocultural approach to Aelius Aristides' *Orationes* and a more thorough exploration of the possibility of Aristides to have had dreams similar to those reported in his work, see Panagiotidou 2019.

desire or wish during dreaming (Holowchak 2002, 159).[24] Furthermore, the oneiric records varied in length and range from detailed descriptions to very brief references. The bizarreness, which characterizes dreams and is totally missing from the healing inscriptions, is an obvious feature in some of Aristides' oneiric records. The content of these tales also ranged from totally bizarre and weird to straight and precise sequences of events. In his dreams, Aristides appears to meet various healing deities, priests, temple servants, friends, eminent people, and even strangers, who participate in the oneiric scenes, which usually take place at the healing sanctuaries and may diverge in theme (Holowchak 2002, 159-160). There are about 60 references to individuals and deities who appeared in Aristides' dreams, among which Asclepius is explicitly referred in three cases. In *Oratio* II 18, Aristides appeared to be at Smyrna, and Asclepius is revealed to him as both himself and Apollo. In III 46, the divine physician along with Isis and Sarapis appears to Aristides at the temple of Isis in Smyrna, and in IV 50, the orator dreams of Asclepius who resembles his statues (Holowchak 2002, 158; cf. *IG* IV(2), 1; Renberg 2010, 36-37; Cilliers and Retief 2013, 78).

All the oneiric tales narrate stories relevant to Aristides' health, and are somehow related to the healing powers of the deities. The treatments employed or prescribed by the divine healers resemble the medical practices of human doctors of the second century CE. They only differ in regard of the conditions under which these treatments are suggested – conditions that the mortal physicians would have considered to be paradoxical or even risky (Holowchak 2002, 158-160).

Based on these observations, Aristides appeared to have self-awareness during dreaming. He was also aware of the phenomenal experience of the objects, other people, and events which comprised the oneiric scene. He was not surprised by the bizarreness of his dreams, the contents of which would have been formed based on his previous knowledge, memories, feelings, and desires. Therefore, I suggest that although Aristides's

---

24. On the potential credibility of Aelius Aristides oneiric reports, see Harris 2009, 118-122; Panagiotidou 2019. For a study of *Orationes* as a product of the wider cultural, intellectual and religious context of its era, see, for example, Petsalis-Diomidis 2010, 122-150. For approaching the *Orationes* as a kind of aretalogy and praise of Asclepius, see, for example, Petsalis-Diomidis 2006; Downie 2013a, 23-35; Petridou 2018. For a psychological interpretation of the dreams of Aelius Aristides, see, for example, Stephens 2012. For the oneiric diary of Aelius Aristides as a literary piece and its connection with the wider life narrative of the orator, see, for example, Downie 2013a. For the readers' embodied perception of the *Orationes*, see Tagliabue 2016.

142 • *The Culmination of Incubation*

oneiric records possibly went through some review after the orator woke up, and perhaps some of their elements were forgotten or eliminated, the *Orationes* could have been quite close to the dreams that he had actually experienced. If this is so, Aelius Aristides' oneiric diary would reflect the ways in which the general settings of the Asclepius cult were inscribed into supplicants' mnemonic systems, and could be recalled and perhaps transformed during their dreams in the *abaton*. Their desire for recovery and residual memories from their strolls within the sanctuary could have modulated the contents of their dreams which would have not been constrained by the physical waking reality. The dreams might include extreme surgical operations and other paradoxical prescriptions given by the god who appeared to use the medical practices of mortal doctors in the weirdest ways. Thus, the surrounding practices and the external representational forms might influence the inner experiences of supplicants, and acquire a subjective, personal expression in their dreams (Graham 1994, 724). And these inner, subjective experiences could be communicated to others through the healing narratives and inscriptions. In this way, the personal healing reported by each supplicant could be evolved to a socially shared experience.[25]

In this view, every healing narrative, inscription, and anatomical votive offering could be perceived as representations of extremely profound personal experiences as well as unique expressions of individual subjectivity. Narrating and inscribing their dreams and healings, supplicants would publicly express their internal experiences rendering them accessible to others. Looking at the inscriptions and hearing personal healing stories, the supplicants collectively experienced what was initially presented as an individual subjective experience of the dreamer. From that moment, these stories did not exclusively belong to the persons who had dreamed them (cf. Graham 1994, 737). They became part of the healing repertoire of the Asclepius cult and could affect and modulate the future dreaming experiences of newcomer supplicants (cf. Ahearne-Kroll 2014a).

In parallel, the fact that the healing narratives and inscriptions were supposed to outline in broad terms supplicants' experiences during incubation, eliminating details and nuances which might derive from individual idiosyncrasies, background life-stories, knowledge, and memories, they left much room for subjective experiences in the *abaton*. The words

---

25. On inner subjectivity and the importance of its public demonstration, see Graham 1994.

dream and *vision* used by the inscriptions regarding the mental conditions of the incubants indicate that their experiences during incubation were supple, and could resemble any kind of altered state of consciousness, ranging from dreaming to hypnotic-like experiences and visionary states. In this way, the wording covered and justified every possible mental reaction of supplicants in the isolated environment of the abaton.

Indirect or Implicit Suggestion: Inducing a Healing Hypnotic-like Experience

Although there is no adequate evidence about what exactly happened in the *abaton* and the precise nature of incubation, the general cult context with the inscriptions, anatomical votive offerings, rituals, and sacrifices as well as the content of these inscriptions, healing narratives, and possible discussions with the priests or other attendants would perhaps operate – as already mentioned – as a form of indirect or implicit suggestion,[26] which could induce a kind of altered state of consciousness in patients resembling therapeutic, hypnotic healing (cf. Cilliers and Retief 2013, 77; Panagiotidou 2021a).

In particular, according to Milton Erickson's model of therapeutic suggestion (Erickson, Rossi and Rossi 1976, 58), 'psychological implication'[27] is a major process through which the patient's 'associative processes' are structured and transformed into 'predictable patterns', without awareness of this transformation (cf. Rossi and Rossi 2007, 268). In this case, although suggestion might implicitly derive from external stimuli – healing narratives, inscriptions, votive offerings, discussions, potential instructions – psychological implications are generated at a subliminal level, automatically activating the subject's cognitive processes and associations, which

---

26. As François Chamoux (2003, 335) has briefly pointed out, 'while medical practice in the Hippocratic tradition was not foreign to the kind of healing that Asclepius provided, it is certain that psychical methods, like autosuggestion, also played a major part in it;' see also Askitopoulou et al. 2002, 4–5; Cilliers and Retief 2013, 86.

27. Erickson, Rossi and Rossi 1976, 58: 'For Erickson, psychological implication is a key that automatically turns the tumblers of a patient's associative processes into predictable patterns without awareness of how it happened. The implied thought or response seems to come up autonomously within patients, as if it were their own inner response rather than a suggestion initiated by the therapist. Psychological implication is thus a way of structuring and directing patients' associative processes when they cannot do it for themselves.'

can induce hypnotic experiences (Erickson, Rossi and Rossi 1976, 59; Rossi and Rossi 2007, 268).

In the wider psychological context of the healing encounter, each patient could perceive him or herself as the focal point, and every condition and experience presented in this context could be consciously or unconsciously taken and transformed to apply to his or her own case (Rossi and Rossi 2007, 269). In this way, psychological implications could indirectly evoke and utilize patient's associations in coping with his or her particular problems (Erickson, Rossi and Rossi 1976, 59–60; Rossi and Rossi 2007, 268). From Ernest and Kathryn Rossi's neuroscience perspective, 'it is the patient's own creative activity that evokes activity – dependent gene expression, brain, and behavioral plasticity, and the so-called "miracles of mind-body healing"' (Rossi and Rossi 2007, 269).

From this point of view, when patients had completed the preparatory rituals and purifications, they entered the *abaton* and stayed there alone in the darkness. In this isolated, perceptually deprived, peaceful atmosphere, the replay of implicit memories, primed images, expectations, suggested information and mental representations reconstructed and re-associated their subjective experiences and could induce a hypnotic-like experience (Panagiotidou 2021a). Having received 'appropriate therapeutic suggestions', which could operate as 'implicit processing heuristics' (Rossi and Rossi 2007, 269), patients possibly activated their own therapeutic resources and self-healing processes to solve their health problems.

An altered state of consciousness, even if it was not a kind of hypnosis in the modern sense of the word, is implied by the very term 'incubation' as well as by the references to states of sleeping and dreaming in the inscriptions (cf. Glicksohn 1991, 1057). Furthermore, the fact that patients should enter in the *abaton* alone and lie down on the ground, expecting to fall asleep and receive a therapeutic dream or vision from Asclepius, probably entailed a kind of hypnotic condition. 'A reduction in sensory stimulation' as a result of isolation and surrounding obscurity, 'a reduction in bodily activity', since patients should stay recumbent on their pallets, and 'a narrowing of attention' are considered to be crucial factors of typical hypnotic conditions, accompanied by 'perceptual deprivation' in the *abaton* (Glicksohn 1991, 1058).

In conditions of perceptual deprivation people may experience various perceptual anomalies as they shift from waking state to sleep and vice versa. Often in this condition, patients do not know with certainty whether they are awake, drowsy, asleep, or dreaming, while they may continually totter between wakefulness, drowsiness and sleep. From a neurophysiological as well as from a subjective perspective, perceptual deprivation phenomena are perceived and conceived of as a kind of 'waking dream' (Glicksohn 1991, 1058; Panagiotidou 2021a). Furthermore, conditions of perceptual deprivation resemble hypnotic induction states and seem to influence and enhance both general and hypnotic suggestibility. In particular, 'hypnagogic-like states' cause 'hyper-suggestibility' which can be further enhanced by the subject's desires and expectations to have unusual, weird, or even numinous experiences (Glicksohn 1991, 1059).

Aristides, in his *Orationes*, mentions a state resembling that of intermediating sleep and waking:

> It [sc. the remedy] was revealed in the clearest way possible, just as countless other things also made the presence of the god manifest. For I seemed almost to touch him and to perceive that he himself was coming, and to be halfway between sleep and waking and to want to get the power of vision and be anxious lest he depart beforehand, and to have turned my ears to listen, sometimes in a dream, sometimes in a waking vision, and my hair was standing on end and tears of joy (came forth), and the weight of knowledge was no burden – what man could even set these things forth in words?
> (Aristid. *Or.* XLVIII, 31–35, trans. Edelstein and Edelstein 1998, T. 417)

In this view, Asclepius' supplicants used to enter the *abaton* seeking a supernatural experience and divine revelation. Probably they were ready to receive any unusual kind of 'cognitive imagery and sensory experiences' (Glicksohn 1991, 1059) occurring there. Seeking extraordinary experiences of divine revelation was possibly attuned and interacted with the ritual environment of the *abaton* that favoured the inducement of altered sensory states rendering patients particularly susceptible to deprivation effects causing experiences in an altered state of consciousness (Glicksohn 1991, 1065).

Embodied Knowledge and Simulation Process: Incubation, Dreams and Visions

The ancient written sources and the inscriptions from the *asclepieia* report that the god used to reveal himself to his supplicants through *dreams* or *visions* during incubation. Iamblichus (*De Mysteriis*, 3, 3, 45) mentions that in the *asclepieia* 'diseases are healed through divine dreams; and, through the order of nocturnal appearances, the medical art is obtained from sacred dreams' (trans. Taylor 1821).

The embodiment theory of religious knowledge, formulated by Laurence Barsalou and his colleagues (2005), would offer valuable insights on the cognitive processes and imagery which could potentially induce divine dreams and visions in Asclepius' supplicants (see Panagiotidou 2021a).

Increasing evidence from cognitive psychology, social psychology and cognitive neuroscience seems to support Barsalou's hypothesis that 'knowledge' – both mundane and religious – 'is grounded in the brain's modality-specific systems' (Barsalou et al. 2005, 19–34; see further Warrington and McCarthy 1987; Damasio 1989; Damasio and Damasio 1994; Pulvermüller 1999; Humphreys and Forde 2001; Martin 2001; Cree and McRae 2003; Simmons and Barsalou 2003). Human beings in their everyday interaction with their surroundings tend to focus on various components of their experiences formulating unconscious 'categorical knowledge about these components' (Barsalou et al. 2005, 15; see further Barsalou 1999, 2003). Repeated focusing 'on a particular component of experience' as well as on certain 'types of settings, events, actions, mental states, properties and relations' entails the establishment of categorical knowledge about these entities and situations (Barsalou et al 2005, 15). This kind of knowledge is encoded, stored in memory systems, and recalled, permeating almost every form of cognitive activity. In particular, the knowledge grounded in the brain's modality-specific systems supports and enhances the perceptual processing of different situations, enabling humans to anticipate events and entities that are likely to be perceived on certain occasions. Perceptions are facilitated and accelerated 'through figure-ground segregation, anticipation, filling in, and other perceptual inferences' (Barsalou et al. 2005, 16).

Furthermore, ordinary knowledge seems to play a crucial role in perceptual processing during offline cognition (e.g. thought, memory, language). In memory, a past event is recalled and becomes a source of speculation and elaborative inferences. In language, words acquire specific meanings and compose phrases and texts conveying ideas, thoughts, and scripts of actual or imagined actions. In thought, objects and events are represented and become objects of reasoning (Barsalou et al. 2005, 16–17; see further Glenberg, Schroeder and Robertson 1998).

However, mundane knowledge is not constrained only to represent, recall, and process already experienced events, situations, and phenomena.

According to Barsalou and his colleagues (2005, 16) 'categorical knowledge' is subsumed and combined with previously acquired and already stored knowledge, and generates simulations of events which can be mentally reactivated in similar contexts. Thus, people are able to visualize and perceive non-present situations, plan their future actions, and generate new concepts and abstract notions. Their perceptual system, establishing mundane knowledge about various components of experiences, can recombine the representations of these components in new ways representing new entities (Barsalou et al. 2005, 17f.; see further Donald 1991; Rips 1995; Hampton 1997; Wisniewski 1997).

Since mundane knowledge influences every form of cognitive activity and processing, it probably seems to penetrate and affect the formulation of religious beliefs and precepts. Usually, people acquire and store specific knowledge about religious institutions, practices, rituals and their meanings (Barsalou et al. 2005, 18). Then they can simulate relevant religious contexts even in their absence or during offline cognition, and can mentally situate themselves in these contexts extracting information from this simulation and forming their subjective experiences (Barsalou et al. 2005, 28). These simulation processes seem to constitute the major cognitive and imaginary mechanism which generates seemingly numinous religious experiences – such as visions – during mundane religious practices – such as prayers and rituals (Barsalou et al. 2005, 36–37). Thus, religious visions seem grounded in the common significant property of human cognition to re-enact and simulate modality-specific states and events that are subjectively experienced and to acquire personal meaning and significance (Barsalou et al. 2005, 36f.).

In this view, the divine healing visions that Asclepius' supplicants claimed to have experienced in the *abaton* might derive from the simulation mechanisms of mundane and religious knowledge – stored and processed in their brain's modality-specific systems – during incubation. A variety of probable sources could induce the content and form of religious visions. In particular, artistic representations of religious figures and events could offer implicit information and knowledge about these entities, which could be re-enacted and simulated later in their absence (Barsalou et al. 2005, 37).

Supplicants, wandering around in the sanctuary, viewed many Asclepius statues and votive relief representations of the patient–god encounters. Particular neural states in their visual systems would represent these images and be taken up by association areas. During incubation, these association areas could re-activate the supplicants' visual system' to partially simulate previously seen images. This activation of their visual systems and subsequent simulations would be enriched by the content of healing narratives which patients had probably heard about or read in the inscriptions before entering the *abaton*. Since people use simulations to represent textual meanings, the perceived words and phrases produce simulations in a similar manner with the icons and pictures which generate visual representations. Thus, the stories and meanings conveyed in the inscriptions would probably be simulated in the modality-specific systems of the supplicants' brains (cf. Barsalou et al. 2005, 38–39).

However, rather than simulating the sculptures, reliefs and stories of the inscriptions as such, patients would subjectively reform their relevant contents and combine simulations in order to represent situations which they had never actually experienced. During incubation, supplicants might vividly simulate the image of Asclepius – as they had viewed him in his sculpture or relief representations – to reveal himself as a vision. Furthermore, they could simulate the main features of the god's encounter with his patients described in the healing narratives, situating themselves in the position of other persons and thus making the experience more personal. In this way, modality-specific representations of the religious content were stored in memory and might be used in the incubation context, thus simulating experiences of personal encounter with the god in the form of divine visions (Barsalou et al. 2005, 38–39).

In this perspective, although divine visions and dreams reported by Asclepius' supplicants after incubation might be perceived as unique and spectacular experiences, they might emerge from the common simulation mechanisms that underlie various cognitive processes and generate the contents of personal dreaming and other imaginative events (Barsalou et al. 2005, 48).

The Day Comes: Reporting the Healing Experience

By sunrise, the ritual of incubation had been accomplished, and the supplicants exited the *abaton*. Those who had experienced a cure or treatment by Asclepius in their sleep should offer thanksgiving and express their gratitude for the successful healing (Von Ehrenheim 2015, 97–111; Renberg 2017, 260–268). The patients who had received prescriptions by the god should follow the divine instructions in order to recover. The incubants who had received a puzzling dream or vision, could classify themselves in lists in order to ask for interpretation by the priests or temple *sacristans* (Nutton 2005, 276; Panagiotidou 2011, 131–132; Von Ehrenheim 2015, 99–101).

Beyond their obligations to Asclepius, exiting the *abaton* the supplicants would probably meet their friends or relatives who might have accompanied them to the sanctuary, and would expect to hear about patients' experiences during incubation. Thus, the incubants were called upon to recall their memories and to describe them to their accompaniers. They would further dictate these memories to the craftsmen who would inscribe them on votive inscriptions.[28]

Thinking, re-thinking, and talking about their experiences in the *abaton* would probably increase the vividness of the described events and would transform them into autobiographical memories (cf. Johnson 2001, 5256). Humans construct these kinds of memories as narratives that situate themselves in a certain place and time and attempt to give meaning to their personal experiences (Johnson 1993, 54–55). And since the human brain continually processes complex information from both external and internal milieus, integrating it in perceivable patterns, it intends to fill in the gaps and attribute coherence to received information (Nichols and Chemel 2006, 25).[29]

Thus, the narratives of autobiographical memories are influenced by the wider context in which they develop, since this context constitutes the tacit natural, cultural, symbolic, and interpersonal background for an individual's self-perception (Johnson 1993, 159). The expectations that people have before the events happen, as well as the reflection after the events and the specific goals and intentions of recollection, can also affect

---

28. On the role that was ascribed to Mnemosyne, the ancient Greek goddess of memory, in the ritual context of the Asclepius cult, for recalling and recording the incubants' dreams, see Ahearne-Kroll 2014b.

29. See the interesting field experiments which confirm my argument about the constructed nature of episodic narratives that was conducted by Dimitris Xygalatas and an international team of colleagues on the San Pedro Manrique firewalking ritual in Spain. They demonstrate that the episodic memories of participants in this high arousal ritual were strongly suppressed immediately after the event, but increased in confidence and detail as time passed. They suggest that 'this mechanism leaves the arousal-induced memory formation empty for cultural schemas and socially negotiated constructions to fill the gap. We suggest that this mechanism may facilitate the construction of a canonical memory of collective rituals that matches the norms and beliefs of a given culture' (Xygalatas et al. 2013, 14; cf. Xygalatas 2012).

the autobiographical memories, attributing to them certain meanings and cohesion. The content of these narratives can also be influenced and even be enriched by similar facts experienced by others (Johnson 2001, 5256). In the Asclepius cult context, such sharing of common experiences among supplicants was achieved through the healing narratives, inscriptions, anatomical votive offerings, and other incubant's accounts.

According to Marcia Johnson, these same processes of association, imagination and reasoning which underlie complex thought and produce true memories can also generate false memories (Johnson 2001).[30] She defines a false memory as 'a mental experience that is mistakenly taken to be a veridical representation of an event from one's personal past' (Johnson 2001, 5254). Such errors mainly derive from the false attribution of an imagined event to actual perception. Humans can subliminally make memory errors while trying to adjust their stories to their own as well as to others' expectations influenced by their wider (cult) contexts (Johnson 2001, 5254). Further beliefs, goals, and motivations as well as social influences, consistency with pre-existing knowledge, coherence of the provided information, and agreement with others' expectations and reports about a certain event can generate a false memory and further embed it in a person's autobiographical narrative. In this process, the mental experiences arising from imagination are imperfectly distinguished from those deriving from actual perception, and are taken as actual memories (Johnson 2001, 5256). This confusion and the conviction that an imagined event actually occurred can be enhanced when the person is called upon to think and talk about this event – a process that can increase the vividness and probability of the imagined experience (Johnson 2001, 5256).

Furthermore, as Nicholas Spanos and his colleagues suggest (1998), memories of imagined extraordinary events can be perceived as actually having happened, when the social context creates relevant expectations in individuals and makes such events particularly plausible and predictable (cf. Johnson 2001, 5257).

In the Asclepius case, the general cult settings presented the appearance of Asclepius in his supplicants' dreams and the performance of divine healings as expectable events. After incubation, the authoritative figures of priests and temple *sacristans* perhaps posed questions to supplicants about their experiences in the *abaton*. Through this questioning,

---

30. On false memories, see Hyman, Husband and Billings 1995; Loftus and Pickrell 1995; Conway 1997; Loftus 1997; Johnson and Raye 1998; Spanos et al. 1998.

they would induce certain imagery to the incubants which could enhance the latter's conviction about the actuality of their healing experiences. Especially the fact that Asclepius' supplicants were inducted into a hypnotic or similar altered state of consciousness in combination with the multiple suggestions derived from their surroundings could induce false memories of their experiences during incubation (Johnson 2001, 5257).[31]

After they waken, perhaps they could recall the oneiric or visionary content of their experiences. Since they could have been repeatedly asked to narrate their dreams or visions, their reports could be organized according to narrative principles, eliminating the inconsistencies and bizarreness and filling the gaps in the oneiric plot. Their narratives would gradually become more detailed, embellished with new representations which might resemble actual perceptions.

Particularly, as Johnson (2001, 5257-5258) suggests, false memories increase when individuals are prompted to embed a certain memory in other supporting details which are relevant to their personal stories. A certain social context can provide the appropriate conditions for 'repeating and embellishing' such memories, encouraging individuals to ignore their doubts and speculations and relax their criteria about the reality of their experiences (Johnson 2001, 5257). And this process is more easily accomplished in the case of 'individuals with high imagery ability' that are 'more susceptible to induced false memories' (Johnson 2001, 5257).

The Asclepius cult seemingly incorporated such features that facilitate false memories. The general cult context comprised a source of information which created certain expectations in the supplicants about what might happen during incubation, used various suggestions in order to make them susceptible to extraordinary experiences, provided them with other people's reports which could embellish the incubant's personal memories, induced certain imagery, and offered the appropriate stimuli for recalling and talking about a patient's experiences in the *abaton*. The supplicants themselves strongly desired to have personal communication with Asclepius who could save them from their sufferings. This desire would make them highly sensitive to every kind of healing experience deriving from reality or imagination, and could interpret even imagined events as actually having happened through 'imperfect reality monitoring processes' (Johnson 2001, 5255). The stories which they narrated after incubation could embed the information derived from the priests'

---

31. On the false memories produced in hypnotic or dissociative states, see Ofshe 1992.

questioning, other people's reports and their own imagination or perceptions. And through repeated recalling, thinking, and narrating, these stories might acquire the quality of autobiographical memories, which might constitute a significant part of the supplicant's life-narratives.

Furthermore, the false memories which supplicants might embed in their healing narratives could derive from their intentions to prove to their relatives, friends, and acquaintances that their decision to visit the *asclepieia*, spending their time and money, was not in vain. Thus, the possibility of cognitive dissonance which could have resulted from their admission of a vacuous decision both to themselves and to others would impel them to proclaim that they had actually found relief from Asclepius (Lyttkens 2011, 21).[32]

Departing from the *asclepieia* and returning to their ordinary lives, patients who had been healed by Asclepius had a personal story to tell to their relatives, friends and acquaintances. This story which would have been perceived and presented as an actual experience might in turn influence other people's beliefs and expectations about the healing powers of the divine physician, generating a continuous flow of supplicants to his temples, who also sought to meet Asclepius, and were eager to interpret their experiences at the sanctuaries as actual evidence of the god's supernatural healing powers.

---

32. On the economics of cognitive dissonance, cf. Akerlof and Dickens 1982.

Conclusion

Completing the Loop

From the Asclepius Cult and the Placebo Effect to Historians and Cognitivists' Consilience

Asclepius evolved to the most renowned healing deity of Graeco-Roman antiquity, and his popularity attracted many supplicants to his sanctuaries. The great *asclepieia* developed into significant healing centres visited by patients seeking recovery.

The purpose of this study was to examine the possibility of the Asclepius cult to provide actual healing experiences to people who suffered from various illnesses and diseases and resorted to the *asclepieia* as supplicants. This examination was built up on historical data about the Asclepius cult and experimental findings of the cognitive sciences, that I applied to the context of this particular historical phenomenon.

The study began from the observations that, according to the ancient testimonies, the Asclepius cult developed into a popular healing cult of the Graeco-Roman world, and cures and treatments were performed at the *asclepieia*. Then I proceeded to examine the hypothesis previously suggested by historians that healing experiences at the Asclepius temples could be generated by supplicants' placebo responses. Therefore, the main question posed was whether there was the possibility for Asclepius supplicants to experience actual health improvement and recovery during their visits at the *asclepieia* as a result of placebo effects.

In order to apply modern cognitive theories to a past religious tradition, the study was based on some major premises. On the one hand, I argued that the external world is governed by certain natural laws which are universal and operate independently of the human agents and, on the other hand, that the human species has developed certain cognitive mechanisms during evolution that enable humans to perceive the world, interact with their surroundings, move around and communicate with each other. These common cognitive abilities enable human agents to attribute meaning to the material world, and to perceive and interpret their surroundings in various ways generating different cultural contexts. These cultural contexts consist of dynamic patterns of practice which are perpetually formed and re-formed through the continual interaction between human neural networks and their external surroundings, transforming these surroundings and re-engineering human cognition.

From this perspective, this study approached the Asclepius cult as a particular pattern of practice which developed in Greek antiquity, flourished in the Graeco-Roman world and finally declined as a result of continual interaction between human agents and their constantly mutating external natural, social and cultural surroundings. Despite the formulation of the major features of the cult in specific historical and cultural settings, however, its success and popularity largely depended on its appeal to major cognitive proclivities and embodied experiences that humans share throughout history. Succumbing to an illness or a disease is a universal human experience that disrupts patients' ordinary lives and well-being, and prompts them to make decisions and take actions in order to restore their health. The wider cultural and social contexts of the ancient Greek world determined the conception of health and illness, and provided a range of choices of which people could make use seeking a cure. In this view, the Asclepius cult emerged as a particular healing option among others comprising the medical pluralism of that era in order to cover the diachronic and universal human need of health and well-being.

Based on these insights, the next stage was the examination of whether the Asclepius cult provided the necessary conditions for inducing placebo responses in the supplicants. Original experimental tests of this hypothesis were not possible, since we could not actually reconstruct the historical contexts of the Asclepius cult in real time, and repeat the experiments in these contexts. However, the study took into consideration the theoretical models and experimental findings of modern studies of the placebo effects, which have determined the parameters and preconditions for placebo responses, and examined whether these parameters and preconditions can be traced in the Asclepius cult. In order to do so, I used the model of placebo effects presented by Humphrey as the wider theoretical framework which I further supported with experimental findings and applied to the cult of Asclepius.

In order to explore how the wider historical, cultural, social and religious contexts of the Graeco-Roman world would have influenced and formed the personal experiences of sickness, I reconstructed the patients' bodily and mental journeys from their homelands to their visits to the *asclepieia* and their cures, as a sequential narrative. Although all patients of the Graeco-Roman era did not follow the same pathways to recovery, this study investigated the potential external influences and internal reactions which could have led at least some of them to resort to the *asclepieia*, appropriating this specific healing option and making them amenable to placebo responses.

In this light, the journeys of Asclepius supplicants to the *asclepieia* were conceived as purposeful enterprises, which began from people's hope for recovery that led them to make the decision to undertake these journeys, and involved their bodily and mental movements along a pathway which would lead them to the planned destination of the Asclepius sanctuaries and hoped-for cure. Since patients' decisions were the starting point of the journey, I explored the external cultural and social influences on their decision-making processes. In particular, the social conditions, cultural influences, religious pursuits and intellectual debates of the Graeco-Roman era were examined which made the visit to the *asclepieia* an attractive choice. The attitudes towards Hippocratic medicine, and the recognition of the Asclepius' authority as a health provider by mortal doctors was suggested as a powerful trigger that encouraged patients to believe in the Asclepian healing power. The healing narratives, circulating among people of the Graeco-Roman world, propagated the effectiveness of Asclepian therapeutic methods, and contributed to the popularity of the cult. In addition, I suggested that the establishment of the Asclepius cult as a healing option in people's minds was enhanced by the observation of other patients who visited the *asclepieia*. Thus, the ideas and beliefs about Asclepius – which diffused through cultural learning, social interactions and interpersonal communication between the people of the Graeco-Roman world – were presented as effective means of formulating patients' choices to ask for his aid. Hope was particularly emphasized as the motivational force that prompted patients to take the decision, and plan their journeys to the *asclepieia*. Since the decision was taken and the itinerary was designed, it was suggested that patients might have experienced an immediate relief from their illnesses as a response to the divine healing prospect.

Arrival at the Asclepius sanctuaries was examined as the next step of patients' journeys to recovery. Focusing on supplicants' arrival at the *asclepieia*, and the time they spent there before the ritual of incubation, the various techniques and means used by the Asclepius cult as well as their impacts on the supplicants' minds and bodies, were examined which could transform patients' hopes into specific expectations of recovery. In the cult context, I outlined how various ordinary experiences would be invested with symbolic and healing qualities, and interpreted as significant divine revelations by supplicants. This ascription of salience to seemingly random events was attributed to high emotional arousal and attention reinforcement during supplicants' participation in the cult practices. Particularly, I examined the impacts of the healing narratives and anatomical votive offerings on the supplicants' reflective beliefs and conformity bias. The healing narratives were approached as a means of indirect suggestion which determined the appropriate behaviour within the sanctuary, and the consequences of anyone breaking the cult rules. These stories also implied the personal responsibility of the patients for their positive health outcomes. The cure was presented as possible only if the patients would adhere to the Asclepian prescriptions and fulfil their vows. In this way, I suggested that the healing narratives could induce self-efficacy expectations in the supplicants. Furthermore, I approached the narratives as effective means of priming specific images and experiences which determined supplicants' expectations of the ritual of incubation. The anatomical votive offerings were also studied as a means of indirect suggestion that encouraged patients to focus on their inflicted body parts, and to expect the application of specific remedies to these parts. I argued that these techniques of priming and suggestion, embedded in the material constructions of the Asclepius cult, could operate to convince supplicants of the healing power of the god, and make them more suggestible to the experiences they were about to have in the *abaton*. Furthermore, the inscriptions and votive offerings were approached as effective means of inducing placebo responses during incubation. According to Humphrey's model, entering the *abaton*, the supplicants were aware that they were going to receive an immediate treatment or a prescription by the god. They believed in these treatments because Asclepius had a universal reputation, testified by the healing narratives and offerings, bearing out the god's authority. Therefore, they could expect that, if they follow the god's instructions, they would be cured. I argued that these expectations *could* later activate their self-healing systems making health improvement possible during incubation.

Regarding the healing narratives in particular, historians have discussed and questioned the credibility of these stories which reported extraordinary treatments. The record of some supplicants' reactions who, as we saw in the fourth chapter, laughed and mocked at the possibility of cure, supports historians' observation that miraculous treatments would have been hard to believe. Neither historians nor supplicants needed to study physics and biology in order to conclude that some of the recorded cures were not only unbelievable but even inconceivable. Such a conclusion derives from a commonsense understanding of the world that is constantly updated through cultural learning. Violations of intuitive and cultural understandings of the world, however, would have different results for historians and supplicants. This difference derives from the fact that the wider social, cultural and religious contexts of the ancient Greek world were different than those of today. Also, supplicants would have had different needs, intentions, desires and expectations than modern historians. While historians attempt to make sense of the past through rationalization, supplicants who lived in the past, shared common perceptions and ideas about perceivable reality, and strived to survive in the adverse conditions caused by illnesses or diseases.

In this light, the people of the ancient Greek world who faced health problems and sought relief, moved by their desire and hope for recovery, would have loosened their rational commonsense understanding of the world, resorting to adaptive errors and allowing cognitive space for violations of commonsense reality. As emphasized by Boyer, religious concepts which minimally violate intuitive human expectations of major ontological categories of the world take people by surprise, grab their attention and become memorable, without demolishing the overall perceivable reality. The violations of shared cultural expectations can have similar effects in attention and memory.

Entering the *abaton*, I suggested that the patients' hopes and expectations of recovery, along with previous conditioning with medical practices, the images primed by the healing narratives and suggestions from the wider cult milieu, would have influenced and shaped the healing experiences of the incubants. I took into account modern research on dreaming, suggestion, and religious visions in order to show how supplicants' residual memories and desires as well as suggested thoughts and imagery could have affected their imagination in the perceptually deprived settings of the *abaton*. While being alone in the darkness, patients' expectations, implicit memories, primed imagery, suggested information and mental representations, supplemented by the wider interpretational background of the Asclepius cult, could re-associate and re-synthesize incubants' subjective experiences, thus inducing an altered state of consciousness resembling hypnosis. In this mental and bodily condition, the simulation mechanisms of the patients' brains could have generated dreams and visions which would be interpreted as divine revelations within the cult context. Thus, I suggested that a placebo drama could unfold in the *abaton*, during which patients, Asclepius, the ritual settings and the therapeutic practices played a crucial role in the healing process. In particular, the emotional, psychological and cognitive conditions of the supplicants, the appearance and behaviour of Asclepius, as well as the applied healing methods and practices during incubation were examined as components of the placebo dramas, which could have generated placebo responses, and thus improve supplicants' health conditions.

Upon sunrise, the ritual of incubation was completed, and incubants exited the *abaton*. Then, they could meet again their friends and relatives who would expect to hear about the patients' experiences during the night. The recounting of the personal healing stories by supplicants might have re-formulated the contents of these stories. In particular, I examined those mental, cognitive, affective and psychological mechanisms that likely operated in supplicants' brains in order to show how the stories about the healing experiences in the *abaton* could have been transformed into autobiographical memories, perceived by supplicants as actually having happened. By leaving the *asclepieia*, the supplicants' journeys came to an end. Possibly the story-telling of their experiences would continue, when they returned home, and perhaps long after. However, what possibly happened afterwards is another story which was beyond the goals of this research.

In broad terms, the purpose of this study was twofold. On the one hand, I investigated how placebo effects could mediate patients' healing experiences at the *asclepieia*. On the other hand, I examined whether the hypotheses and experimental findings of cognitive studies on placebo effects are supported by historical evidence, and provide valuable explanations of universal human behaviours. In this way, this case-study of the Asclepius cult intends to provide an exemplar of how historical research and cognitive sciences can cooperate, with mutual benefits for both fields.

Cognitive approaches to historical institutions, practices and events bring to the fore human agency in history. The cognitive sciences may provide historians with theoretical frameworks and methodological tools in order to gain a deeper understanding of the human agents who lived in past eras and interacted with their external surroundings. Historians are able to use these tools in order to seek answers to the historical questions they pose. An understanding of human cognition may offer valuable insights into people's motivations, thoughts, reactions, and constructions throughout history, and shed light on the ways in which the meaningful material world influenced people's perceptions, beliefs, attitudes and behaviours, generating multiple patterns of practice.

Particularly in the study of religious healing practices, like the Asclepius cult, the application of cognitive theories could offer a valuable theoretical framework in order to examine the possibility of such practices to have actual health benefits. In addition, the investigation of common cognitive and psychological processes – which move people to look for alternative solutions in order to find relief from their pains, to hope for salvation and to enhance the effectiveness of the applied healing methods through their own self-healing mechanisms – offer new possibilities to historians to examine important questions about, for example, the social interactions that mediated the appearance, flourishing and popularity of these practices, the reasons for their declines and alterations throughout history as well as people's reasoning and beliefs in supernatural healing. Understanding human cognition may further reveal the mechanisms of historical change and the diversity of multiple cultural and social expressions and institutions developed in different places and historical periods.

In parallel, historical studies offer a wider field for cognitive sciences to test the findings of modern experimental and anthropological research. The application of cognitive theories to past practices and behaviours may highlight the ways in which history permeates human cognition. Since humans are, besides embrained and embodied, deeply encultured beings (cf. Geertz 2010), and their cognitive and psychological processes are not restricted in the brain, the examination of various practices and expressions throughout human history can trace the ways in which the external natural, historical, cultural and social settings *re-engineer* the human mind, and may change its perceptual, cognitive and affective abilities.

In the study of the placebo effects, the application of modern theories to the healing cults and religious practices, which flourished in different historical periods, may offer further evidence to support or oppose hypotheses and experimental findings. The studies of placebo effects explore the brain and body mechanisms and processes which generate placebo responses. The external settings, social interactions and individual reactions to various stimuli mediate the activation of these mechanisms. Therefore, a diachronic examination of the conditions and external parameters for the inducement of placebo effects within various historical contexts may offer new evidence and lead to enrichment or improvement of the hypotheses.

From this perspective, a consilience between historical research and the cognitive sciences would promote their common interest in the human mind. Humans as historical agents should be taken into account in the study of human cognition. And it is crucial for the advance of this study that historians participate in the wider interdisciplinary discussions and projects of the cognitive sciences. Towards this end, *cognitive historiography* arose as a much promising field of research. Researchers with a special interest in the human mind investigate how cognitive theories and methods may support historical research and vice versa. Although this endeavour is still at its beginnings, the discussions taking place between historians and cognitive scientists are fruitful, crossing the borders between the disciplines.

Historians are now able to write the history of past human agents based on the primary and secondary sources, and further to support or to disconfirm their commonsense assumptions and interpretations using a valuable and continually growing corpus of knowledge, methods and theories provided by the cognitive sciences. Thus, the application of scientific methods in history is not interdictory. On the contrary, it can be useful and very valuable, if it is used in the service of specific historical quests. All that is needed are questions for research posed by historians.

References

Abbreviations

CIG = *Corpus Inscriptionum Graecorum*
ICr = *Inscriptiones Creticae*
IG = *Inscriptiones Graecae* (1873–)
IG II(2) = *Inscriptiones Graecae* II(2)
IG IV(2), 1, 121–122 = *Inscriptiones Graecae* IV(2), 1, nos 121–122
ILAfr. 225 = *Inscriptions latines d'Afrique*
IPerg. = *Inscriptiones Pergamenae*
LIMC = *Lexicon Iconographicum Mythologiae Classicae*
SEG 20. 759. = Balagrae (El Beida). *Lex sacra*, s. III/IVp. (20–759)

Other references

Abi-Dargham, A., Rodenhiser, J., Printz, D., Zea-Ponce, Y. et al. (2000), 'Increased baseline occupancy of D_2 receptors by dopamine in schizophrenia'. *Proceedings of the National Academy of Sciences of the United States of America* 97 (14), 8104–8109.

Adams, C. D. (ed. and trans.) (1868), *The Genuine Works of Hippocrates by Hippocrates*. New York: Dover.

Ader, R. (1997), 'The role of conditioning in pharmacotherapy'. In A. Harrington (ed.), *The Placebo Effect: An Interdisciplinary Exploration.* (Mind/Brain/Behavior Initiative 8). Cambridge, MA: Harvard University Press, pp. 138–165.

Ader, R., and Cohen, N. (1975), 'Behaviorally conditioned immunosuppression'. *Psychosomatic Medicine* 37, 333–340.

Ader, R., and Cohen, N. (1985), 'CNS–immune system interactions: Conditioning phenomena'. *Behavioral and Brain Sciences* 8 (3), 379–395.

Ader, R., N. Cohen, and D. Felten (1995), 'Psychoneuroimmunology: Interactions between the nervous system and the immune system'. *The Lancet* 345 (8942), 99–103.

Afonasin, E. (2019), 'Neoplatonic Asclepius'. In J. F. Finamore and T. Nejeschleba (eds), *Platonism and its Legacy. Selected Papers from the Fifteenth Annual Conference of the International Society for Neoplatonic Studies*. Lydney: Prometheus Trust, pp. 159–172.

Agras, W. S., Horne, M., and Taylor, C. B. (1982), 'Expectation and the blood-pressure-lowering effects of relaxation'. *Psychosomatic Medicine* 44, 389–395.

Ahearne-Kroll, S. (2014a). 'The afterlife of a dream and the ritual system of the Epidauran asklepieion'. *Archiv für Religionsgeschichte* 15, 35–52.

Ahearne-Kroll, S. (2014b), 'Mnemosyne at the Asklepieia'. *Classical Philology* 109, 99–118.

Akerlof, G. A., and Dickens, W. T. (1982), 'The economic consequences of cognitive dissonance'. *American Economic Review* 72 (3), 307–319.

Aleshire, B. S. (1989), *The Athenian Asklepieion: The People, Their Dedications and The Inventories*. Amsterdam: J. C. Gieben.

Alvarez-Buyalla, R., and Carrasco-Zanini, J. (1960), 'A conditioned reflex which reproduces the hypoglycemic effect of insulin'. *Acta Physiologica Latino Americana* 10, 153–158.

Alvarez-Buyalla, R., Segura, E. T., and Alvarez-Buyalla, E. R. (1961), 'Participation of the hypophysis in the conditioned reflex which reproduces the hypoglycemic effect of insulin'. *Acta Physiologica Latino Americana* 11, 113–119.

Amigo, I., Cuesta, V., Fernández, A., and González, A. (1993), 'The effect of verbal instructions on blood pressure measurement'. *Journal of Hypertension* 11, 293–296.

Amundsen, W. D. (1977), 'Images of the physician in Classical Time'. *Journal of Popular Culture* 11, 643–655.

Amundsen, W. D. (1996), *Medicine, Society, and Faith in the Ancient and Medical Worlds*. Baltimore, MD: Johns Hopkins University Press.

Androutsos, G., Diamantis, A., Vladimiros, L., and Magiorkinis, E. (2008), 'Health and disease in ancient Greek medicine'. *International Journal of Health Science* 2 (1), 20–24.

Antoniou, S. A., Antoniou, G. A., Learney, R., Granderath, F. A., and Antoniou, A. I. (2011), 'The rod and the serpent: History's ultimate healing symbol'. *World Journal of Surgery* 35 (1), 217–221. https://doi.org/10.1007/s00268-010-0686-y

Antrobus, J. S. (1990), 'Neurocognition of sleep mentation: Rapid eye movements, visual imagery, and dreaming'. In R. R. Bootzin, J. F. Kihlstrom and D. L. Schacter (eds), *Sleep and Cognition*. Washington, DC: American Psychological Association, pp. 3–24.

Archer, T. P., and Leier, C. V. (1992), 'Placebo treatment in congestive heart failure'. *Cardiology* 81 (2–3), 125–133.

Ariely, D. (2008), *Predictably Irrational: The Hidden Forces that Shape our Decisions*. New York: HarperCollins.

Arnott, R. (1996), 'Healing and medicine in the Aegean Bronze Age'. *Historical Review* 89, 265–270.

Arnott, R. (2004), 'Minoan and Mycenaean medicine and its Near Eastern contacts'. In H. F. J. Horstmanshoff and M. Stol (eds), *Magic and Rationality in Ancient Near Eastern and Graeco-Roman Medicine.* (Studies in Ancient Medicine 27). Leiden: Brill, pp. 153–173.

Askitopoulou, H., Konsolaki, E., Ramoutsaki, I. A., and Anastassaki, M. (2002), 'Surgical cures under sleep induction in the asclepieion of Epidaurus'. In J. C. Diaz, A. Franco, D. R. Bacon, J. Rupreht and J. Alvarez (eds), *The History of Anesthesia.* (Excerpta Medical International Congress Series 1242). Amsterdam: Elsevier, pp. 11–17.

Asmar, R., Safar, M., and Queneau, P. (2001), 'Evaluation of the placebo effect and reproducibility of blood pressure measurement in hypertension'. *American Journal of Hypertension* 14 (6 Pt 1), 546–552.

Avalos, H. (1995), *Illness and Health Care in the Ancient Near East: The Role of the Temple in Greece, Mesopotamia, and Israel*. Atlanta, GA: Scholars Press.

Babbitt, F. C. (trans.) (1936), Lucius Mestrius Plutarchus, *Moralia*. Cambridge, MA: Harvard University Press.

Baker, P. (2017), 'Viewing health: Asclepia in their natural settings'. *Religion in the Roman Empire* 3 (2), 243–163.

Baloyannis, S. J. (2016), 'Galen as neuroscientist and veurophilosopher'. *Encephalos* 53, 1–10.

Bandura, A. (1997), *Self-efficacy: The Exercise of Control*. New York: Freeman.

Bargh, J. (1997), 'The automaticity of everyday life'. In R. S. Wyer (ed.), *The Automaticity of Everyday Life*. (Advances in Social Cognition Series 10). Mahwah, NJ: Psychology Press, pp. 1–61.

Barsalou, L. W. (1999), 'Perceptual symbol systems'. *Behavioral and Brain Sciences* 22, 577–660.

Barsalou, L. W. (2003), 'Abstraction in perceptual symbol systems'. *Philosophical Transactions of the Royal Society of London: Biological Sciences* 358, 1177–1187.

Barsalou, L. W., Barbey, A. K., Simmons W. K., and Santos, A. (2005), 'Embodiment in religious knowledge'. *Journal of Cognition and Culture* 5 (1–2), 14–57.

Bass M. J., Buck, C., Turner, L., Dickie, G., Pratt, G., and Robinson, H. C. (1986), 'The physician's actions and the outcome of illness in family practice'. *The Journal of Family Practice* 23, 43–47.

Baumgart, H. (1874), *Aelius Aristides als Repräsentant der Sophistischen Rhetorik des Zweiten Jahrhunderts der Kaiserzeit*. Leipzig: Teubner.

Bean, E. G. (1979), *Aegean Turkey*. London: John Murray.

Beard, M. (1986), 'Cicero and divination: The formation of a Latin discourse'. *Journal of Roman Studies* 76, 33–46.

Beck, R. (2014), '"Star-Talk": A gateway to mind in the ancient world'. *Journal of Cognitive Historiography* 1 (1), 90–97.

Beckham, E. E. (1989), 'Improvement after evaluation in psychotherapy of depression: Evidence of a placebo effect?'. *Journal of Clinical Psychology* 45 (6), 945–950.

Beekes, R. S. P. (2009), *Etymological Dictionary of Greek*. Leiden: Brill.

Beerden, K. (2013), *World Full of Signs: Ancient Greek Divination in Context.* (Religions in the Roman World 176). Leiden: Brill.

Behr, A. C. (1968), *Aelius Aristides and the Sacred Dream*. Amsterdam: A. M. Hakkert.

Bekoff, M., Allen, C., and Burghardt, G. (2002), *The Cognitive Animal: Empirical and Theoretical Perspectives on Animal Cognition*. Cambridge, MA: MIT Press.

Bendlin, A. (2007), 'Purity and pollution'. In D. Ogden (ed.), *A Companion to Greek Religion.* (Blackwell Companions to the Ancient World). Oxford: Wiley-Blackwell, pp. 178–189.

Benedetti, F. (2009), *Placebo Effects. Understanding the Mechanisms in Health and Disease*. New York: Oxford University Press.

Benedetti, F., and Amanzio, M. (2011), 'The placebo response: How words and rituals change the patient's brain'. *Patient Education and Counseling* 84 (3), 413–419.

Benedetti, F., Amanzio, M., Casadio, C., Oliaro, A., and Maggi G. (1997), 'Blockade of nocebo hyperlagesia by the cholecystokinin antagonist proglumide'. *Pain* 71 (2), 135–140.

Benedetti, F., Amanzio, M., Vighetti, S., and Asteggiano, G. (2006), 'The biochemical and neuroendocrine bases of the hyperalgesic nocebo effect'. *Journal of Neuroscience* 26, 12,014–12,022.

Benedetti, F., Carlino, E., and Pollo, A. (2011), 'How placebos change the patient's brain'. *Neuropsychopharmacology* 36, 339–354. Retrieved from www.ncbi.nlm.nih.gov/pmc/articles/PMC3055515 (accessed 25 August 2013).

Benedetti, F., Colloca, L., Torre, E., Lanotte, Melcarne, A., Pesare, M., Bergamasco, B., and Lopiano, L. (2004), 'Placebo-responsive Parkinson patients show decreased activity in single neurons of subthalamic nucleus'. *Nature Neuroscience* 7 (6), 587–588.

Benedetti, F., Lanotte, M., Lopiano, L., and Colloca, L. (2007), 'When words are painful: Unraveling the mechanisms of the nocebo effect'. *Neuroscience* 147, 260–271.

Benedetti, F., Mayberg, H. S., Wager, T. D., Stohler, C. S., and Zubieta J. K. (2005), 'Neurobiological mechanisms of the placebo effect'. *Journal of Neuroscience* 25 (45), 10,390–10,402.

Benedetti, F., Pollo, A., Lopiano, L., Lanotte, Vighetti, M. S., and Rainero, I. (2003), 'Conscious expectation and unconscious conditioning in analgesic motor and hormonal placebo/nocebo responses'. *Journal of Neuroscience* 23 (10), 4315–4323.

Benson, H., and Epstein, M. D. (1975), 'The placebo effect: A neglected asset in the care of patients'. *Journal of the American Medical Association* 232 (12), 1225–1227.

Berger, E. (1970), *Das Basler Artzrelief. Studien zum griechischen Grab- und Votivrelief um 500 v. Chr. und zur vorhippokratischen Medizin*. Basel: Archäologischer Verlag/Mainz, von Zabern.

Bering, J., McLeod, K., and Shackelford, T. K. (2005), 'Reasoning about dead agents reveals possible adaptive trends'. *Human Nature* 16 (4), 360–381.

Berlim, M. T., and Abeche, A. M. (2001), 'Evolutionary approach to medicine'. *Southern Medical Journal* 94 (1), 26–32.

Berridge, K. C., and Robinson, T. E. (1998), 'What is the role of dopamine in reward: Hedonic impact, reward learning, or incentive salience?'. *Brain Research Reviews* 28, 309–369.

Beumer, M. (2016), 'Hygieia. Identity, cult and reception'. *Kleio-Historia* 3, 5–24.

Billows, R. (2005), 'Cities'. In A. Erskine (ed.), *A Companion to the Hellenistic World*. (Blackwell Companions to Ancient History). Oxford: Wiley –Blackwell, pp. 196–215.

Błaśkiewicz, M. (2014), 'Healing dreams at Epidaurus. Analysis and interpretation of the Epidaurian iamata'. *Miscellanea Anthropologica et Sociologica* 15 (4), 54–69.

Blum, L. H. (1985), 'Beyond medicine: Healing power in the doctor–patient relationship'. *Psychological Reports* 57, 399–427.

Böck, B. (2014), *The Healing Goddess Gula: Towards an Understanding of Ancient Babylonian Medicine*. Leiden: Brill.

Bonnechere, P. (2007), 'Divination'. In D. Odgen (ed.), *A Companion to Greek Religion*. (Blackwell Companions to the Ancient World). Malden, MA: Blackwell, pp. 145–159.

Bootzin, R. R., and Caspi, O. (2002), 'Explanatory mechanisms for placebo effects: Cognition, personality and social learning'. In H. A. Guess, A. Kleinman, J. W. Kusek and L. W. Engel (eds), *The Science of the Placebo: Toward an Interdisciplinary Research Agenda*. London: BMJ Books, pp. 108–132.

Borkovec, T. D. (1985), 'Placebo: Redefining the unknown'. In L. White, B. Tursky and G. E. Schwartz (eds), *Placebo: Theory, Research and Mechanisms*. New York: Guilford Press, pp. 59–66.

Bostock, J., and Riley, H. T. (trans.) (1855), *The Natural History of Pliny*. London: Henry G. Bohn, MDCCCLV-MDCCCLVII.

Boyer, P (1996), 'What makes anthropomorphism natural: Intuitive ontology and cultural representations'. *The Journal of the Royal Anthropological Institute* 2(1): 83–97. https://doi.org/10.2307/3034634

Boyer, P. (2002), *Religion Explained: The Human Instincts That Fashion Gods, Spirits and*

Ancestors. London: William Heinemann.

Boys-Stones, G. R. (2018), *L. Annaeus Cornutus: Greek Theology, Fragments and Testimonia*. Atlanta, GA: SBL Press.

Braun, A. R., Balkin, T. J., Wesensten, N. J., Gwadry, F. et al. (1998), 'Dissociated pattern of activity in visual cortices and their projections during human rapid eye-movement sleep'. *Science* 279 (5347), 91–95.

Bremmer, J. N. (1981), 'Greek hymns'. In H. S. Versnel (ed.), *Faith, Hope and Worhsip*. Leiden: Brill, pp. 193–215.

Bremmer, J. N. (1994), *Greek Religion*. Oxford: Oxford University Press.

Breznitz, S. (1999), 'The effect of hope on pain tolerance'. *Social Research* 66, 629–652.

Brody, H. (1982) 'The lie that heals: The ethics of giving placebos'. *Annals of Internal Medicine* 97, 112–118.

Brody, H. (1985), 'Placebo effect: An examination of Grunbaum's definition'. In L. White, B. Tursky and G. E. Schwartz (eds), *Placebo: Theory, Research and Mechanisms*. New York: Guilford Press, pp. 37–58.

Brody, H. (2000) 'The placebo response'. *Journal of Family Practice* 49, 649–654.

Brody, H., and Brody, D. (2000), 'Three perspectives on the placebo response: Expectancy, conditioning, and meaning'. *Advances in mind-body medicine* 16, 216–232.

Broom, D. M. (1998), 'Welfare, stress and the evolution of feelings'. *Advances in the Study of Behavior* 27, 371–403.

Broom, D. M. (2001), 'The evolution of pain'. In L. Soulsby and D. Morton (eds), *Pain: Its Nature and Management in Man and Animals. Proceedings of symposium*. Fund for the Replacement of Animals in Medical Research (FRAME). The Royal Society of Medicine. March 2000. London: Royal Society of Medicine Press, pp. 17–25.

Buckman, R., and Sabbagh, K. (1993), *Magic or Medicine: An Investigation of Healing and Healers*. London: MacMillan.

Bulbulia, J. (2006), 'Nature's medicine: Religiosity as an adaptation for health and cooperation'. In P. McNamara (ed.), *Where God and Science Meet. How Brain and Evolutionary Studies Alter Our Understanding of Religion*, vol. 1: *Evolution, Genes and the Religious Brain*. (Psychology, Religion and Spirituality). Westport, CT: Praeger Publishing, pp. 87–121.

Buraselis, K. (2000), *Kos between Hellenism and Rome: Studies on the Political, Institutional and Social History of Kos from ca. the Middle Second Century B.C. Until Late Antiquity*. (Transactions of the American Philosophical Society New Series 90, 4). Philadelphia, PA: American Philosophical Society. https://doi.org/10.2307/1586017

Burford, A. (1969), *The Greek Temple Builders at Epidaurus*. Liverpool: Liverpool University Press.

Burkert, W. (1983), 'Itinerant diviners and magicians: A neglected element in cultural contacts'. In R. Hägg (ed.), *The Greek Renaissance of the Eighth Century B.C.: Tradition and Innovation*. Second International Symposium. Swedish Institute, Athens, 1–5 June 1981. (Acta Instituti Atheniensis Regni Sueciae. Series in 4o). Stockholm: Aströms, pp. 115–119.

Burkert, W. (1985), *Greek Religion*. Cambridge, MA: Harvard University Press.

Burkert, W. (1992), *The Orientalizing Revolution: Near Eastern Influence on Greek Culture in the Early Archaic Age*. Cambridge, MA: Harvard University Press.

Burkert, W. (1994), 'Olbia and Apollo of Didyma: A new oracle text'. In J. Solomon (ed.), *Apollo: Origins and Influences*. London: The University of Arizona Press, pp. 49–60.

Burnett, O. L. (2015), 'The Religion in medicine: An exploration of healing through the examination of Asclepius and the Epidaurian Iamata'. *Prandium: The Journal of Historical Studies* 4 (1), 2–7.

Campbell-Meiklejohn, D. K., Bach, D. R., Roepstorff, A., Dolan, R. J., and Frith, C. D. (2010), 'How the opinion of others affects our valuation of objects'. *Current Biology* 20, 1165–1170.

Carleton, R. N. (2016a), 'Into the unknown: A review and synthesis of contemporary models involving uncertainty'. *Journal of Anxiety Disorders* 39, 30–43. https://doi.org/10.1016/j.janxdis.2016.02.007.

Carleton, R. N. (2016b), 'Fear of the unknown: One fear to rule them all?'. *Journal of Anxiety Disorders* 41, 5–21. http://doi.org/10.1016/j.janxdis.2016.03.011

Cassell, E. J. (1976), *The Healer's Art: A New Approach to the Doctor-Patient Relationship*. Philadelphia, PA: Lippincott.

Cassell, E. J. (1982), 'The nature of suffering and the goals of medicine'. *The New England Journal of Medicine* 306 (11), 639–645.

Cassell, E. J. (1991), *The Nature of Suffering and the Goals of Medicine*. Oxford: Oxford University Press.

Chalupa, A. (2014), 'Pythiai and inspired divination in the Delphic Oracle: Can cognitive sciences provide us with an access to "Dead Minds"?' *Journal of Cognitive Historiography* 1 (1), 24–51.

Chamoux, F. (2003), *Hellenistic Civilization*. Translated by M. Roussel. Oxford: Blackwell.

Chaput de Saintonge, M., and Herxheimer, A. (1994), 'Harnessing placebo effects in healthcare'. *Lancet* 344, 995–998.

Charitonidou, A. (1973), 'Epidaurus: The sanctuary of Asclepius'. In E. Melas (ed.), *Temples and Sanctuaries of Ancient Greece*. London: Thames and Hudson, pp. 89–100.

Christopoulou-Aletra, H., Togia, A., and Varlami, C. (2010), 'The "smart" Asclepieion: A total healing environment'. *Archives of Hellenic Medicine* 27 (2): 259–263.

Churchland, P. (1979), *Scientific Realism and the Plasticity of Mind*. New York: Cambridge University Press.

Churchland, P. (1981), 'Eliminative materialism and the propositional attitudes', *Journal of Philosophy* 78, 67–90.
Churchland, P. (1984), *Matter and Consciousness*. Bradford, MA: MIT Press.
Cicogna, P., and Bosinelly, M. (2001), 'Consciousness during dreaming'. *Consciousness and Cognition* 10, 26–41.
Cilliers, L., and Retief, F. P. (2005), 'Snake and staff symbolism in healing'. *Acta Theologica* (Suppl. 7), 189–199.
Cilliers, L., and Retief, F. P. (2013), 'Dream healing in asclepieia in the Mediterranean'. In S. M. Oberhelman (ed.), *Dreams, Healing, and Medicine in Greece: From Antiquity to the Present*. Farnham: Ashgate, pp. 69–93.
Clark, A. (1997), *Being There: Putting Brain, Body and World Together Again*. Cambridge MA: MIT Press.
Clark, A. (2008), *Supersizing the Mind: Embodiment, Action, and Cognitive Extension*. New York: Oxford University Press.
Coarelli, F. (1987), *I Santuari del Lazio in età repubblicana*. Rome: La Nuova Italia Scientifica.
Cohen, G. M. (1995), *The Hellenistic Settlements in Europe, the Islands, and Asia Minor*. (Hellenistic Culture and Society 17). Berkeley, CA: University of California Press.
Cohn-Haft, L. (1956), *The Public Physicians of Ancient Greece*. Northampton, MA: Smith College.
Colloca, L., and Benedetti, F. (2006), 'How prior experience shapes placebo analgesia'. *Pain* 124 (1), 126–123.
Colloca, L., and Benedetti, F. (2007), 'Nocebo hyperalgesia: How anxiety is turned into pain'. *Current Opinion in Anaesthesiology* 20, 435–439.
Colloca, L., and Benedetti, F. (2009), 'Placebo analgesia induced by social observational learning'. *Pain* 144, 28–34.
Colloca, L., and Miller, F. G. (2011), 'How placebo responses are formed: A learning perspective'. *Philosophical Transactions of the Royal Society B* 366 (1572), 1859–1869.
Colloca, L., Petrovic, P., Wager, T. D., Ingvar, M., and Benedetti F. (2010), 'How the number of learning trials affects placebo and nocebo responses'. *Pain* 151, 430–439.
Colloca, L., Sigaudo, M., and Benedetti, F. (2008a), 'The role of learning in nocebo and placebo effects'. *Pain* 136, 211–218.
Colloca, L., Tinazzi, M., Recchia, S., Le Pera, D., Fiaschi, A., Benedetti, F., and Valeriani, M. (2008b), 'Learning potentiates neurophysiological and behavioral placebo analgesic responses'. *Pain* 139, 306–314.
Combs, A., and Krippner, S. (1998), 'Dream sleep and waking reality: A dynamical view of two states of consciousness'. In S. Hameroff, A. W. Kaszniak and A. C. Scott (eds), *Toward a Science of Consciousness: The Second Tucson Discussions and Debates*. Cambridge, MA: MIT Press, pp. 478–493.

Compton, M. T. (2002), 'The association of Hygieia with Asklepios in Graeco-Roman asclepeio medicine'. *Journal of the History of Medicine and Allied Sciences* 57 (3), 312–339.

Constantino, J. M., Glass, R. C., Arnkoff, B. D., Ametrano, M. R., and Smith, J. Z. (2011), 'Expectations'. *Journal of Clinical Psychology: in session* 67 (2), 184–192. https://doi.org/10.1002/jclp.20754.

Conway, M. A. (ed.) (1997) *Recovered Memories and False Memories*. Oxford: Oxford University Press.

Conybeare, F. C. (trans.) (1912), *The life of Apollonius of Tyana, the Epistles of Apollonius and the Treatise of Eusebius*. New York: G. P. Putnam's Sons.

Cotsapas, C., and Hafler, D. A. (2013), 'Immune-mediated disease genetics: The shared basis of pathogenesis'. *Trends in Immunology* 34 (1), 22–26.

Cotter, W. (1999), *Miracles in Greco-Roman Antiquity*. London: Routledge.

Crawford, M. H., Keppie, L., Patterson, J., and Verenocke, M. L. (1986), 'Excavations at Fregellae, 1978–1984 (part III)'. *Papers of the British School at Rome* 54, 40–68.

Cree, G. S., and K. McRae (2003), 'Analyzing the factors underlying the structure and computation of the meaning of chipmunk, cherry, chisel, cheese, and cello (and many other such concrete nouns)'. *Journal of Experimental Psychology: General* 132 (2), 163–201.

Crick, F., and Koch, C. (1995), 'Are we aware of neural activity in primary visual cortex?'. *Nature* 375, 121–123.

Crow R., Gage, H., Hampson, S., Hart, J., Kimber, A., and Thomas, H. (1999), 'The role of expectancies in the placebo effect and their use in the delivery of health care: A systematic review'. *Health Technology Assessment Journal* 3 (3), 1–96.

Crowe McCann, C., Goldfarb, B., Frisk, M., Quera-Salva, M. A., and Meyer, P. (1992), 'The role of personality factors and suggestion in placebo effect during mental stress test'. *British Journal of Clinical Pharmacology* 33, 107–110.

Csepregi, I. (2011), 'Disease, death, destiny: The healer as soter in miraculous cures'. In C. Krötzl and K. Mustakallio (eds), *On Old Age: Approaching Death in Antiquity and the Middle Ages*. Turnhout: Brepols Publishers, pp. 253–276.

Czajkowski, S. M., and Chesney, M. A. (1990), 'Adherence and the placebo effect'. In S. A. Shumaker, E. B. Schron and J. K. Ockene (eds), *The Handbook of Health Behavior Change*. New York: Springer, pp. 515–534.

Czerniak, E., and Davidson, M. (2012), 'Placebo, a historical perspective'. *European Neuropsychopharmacology* 22 (11), 770–774.

Damasio, A. R. (1989), 'Time-locked multiregional retroactivation: A systems-level proposal for the neural substrates of recall and recognition'. *Cognition* 33, 25–62.

Damasio, A. R., and Damasio, H. (1994), 'Cortical systems for retrieval of concrete knowledge: The convergence zone framework'. In C. Koch and J. L. Davis (eds), *Large-scale Neuronal Theories of the Brain: Computational Neuroscience.* (Computational Neuroscience Series). Cambridge, MA: MIT Press, pp. 61–74.

Daruna, J. H. (2012 [2004]), *Introduction to psychoneuroimmunology*. London: Elsevier Academic Press.

Day, M. (2004), 'Religion, off-line cognition and the extended mind'. *Journal of Cognition and Culture* 4 (1), 101–121.

De Craen, A. J., Kaptchuk, T. J. Tijssen, J. G., and Kleijnen J. (1999a), 'Placebos and placebo effects in medicine: Historical overview'. *Journal of the Royal Society of Medicine* 92 (10), 511–515.

De Craen, A. J. M, Moerman, D. E., Heisterkamp, S. H., Tytgat, G. N. J., Tijssen, J. G., and Kleijnen, J. (1999b), 'Placebo effect in the treatment of duodenal ulcer'. *British Journal of Clinical Pharmacology* 48 (6), 853–860. https://doi.org/10.1046/j.1365-2125.1999.00094.x

Deeley, Q. P. (2004), 'The religious brain: Turning ideas into convictions'. *Anthropology and Medicine* 11 (3), 245–267. https://doi.org/10.1080/1364847042000296554

De la Fuente-Fernández, R., and Stoessl, A. J. (2002a), 'The placebo effect in Parkinson's disease'. *Trends in Neurosciences* 25 (6), 302–306.

De la Fuente-Fernández, R., Phillips, A. F., Zamburlini, M., Sossi, V., Calne, D. B, Ruth, T. J., and Stoessl, A. J. (2002b), 'Dopamine release in human ventral striatum and expectation of reward'. *Behavioral Brain Research* 96, 393–402.

De la Fuente-Fernández, R., Ruth, T. J., Sossi, V., Schulzer, M., Calne, D. B, and Stoessl, A. J. (2001), 'Expectation and dopamine release: Mechanisms of the placebo effect in Parkinson's disease'. *Science.* 293, 1164–1166.

Demand, N. (1994), *Birth, Death, and Motherhood in Classical Greece.* Baltimore, MD: Johns Hopkins University Press.

Denyer, N. (1985), 'The case against divination: An examination of Cicero's *de Divinatione*'. *Proceedings of the Cambridge Philological Society* 211, n.s. 31, 1–10.

Deubner, L. (1900), *De Incubatione Capita Quattuor Scripsit Ludovicus Deubner: Accedit Laudatio in Miracula Sancti Hieromartyris Therapontis E Codice Messanensi Denuo Edita.* Nabu Press.

Deubner, O. (1938), *Das Asclepeio von Pergamon.* Berlin: Verl. f. Kunstwiss.

Di Blasi, Z., Harkness, E., Ernst, E., Georgiou, A., and Kleijnen, J. (2001), 'Influence of context effects on health outcomes: A systematic review'. *Lancet* 357, 757–762. https://doi.org/10.1016/s0140-6736(00)04169-6

Dickie, M. W. (2001), *Magic and Magicians in the Greco-Roman World.* London: Routledge.

Dickie, M. W. (2010), 'Magic in Classical and Hellenistic Greece'. In D. A. Odgen (ed.), *A Companion to Greek Religion.* (Blackwell Companions to the Ancient World). Malden, MA: Wiley-Blackwell, pp. 357–370.

Diener, H. C., Schorn, C. F., Bingel, U., and Dodick, D. W. (2008), 'The importance of placebo in headache research'. *Cephalalgia* 28 (10), 1003–1011.

Dignas, B. (2007), 'A day in the life of a Greek sanctuary'. In D. A. Ogden (ed.), *A Companion to Greek Religion*. (Blackwell Companions to the Ancient World). Malden, MA: Wiley-Blackwell, pp. 163–177.
Dillon, M. P. J. (1994), 'The didactic nature of the Epidaurian iamata'. *Zeitschrift für Papyrologie und Epigraphik* 101, 239–260.
Dillon, M. P. J. (1997), *Pilgrims and Pilgrimage in Ancient Greece*. New York: Routledge.
Dillon, M. P. J. (2002), *Girls and Women in Classical Greek Religion*. New York: Routledge.
Dodds, E. R. (1965), *Pagan and Christian in an Age of Anxiety*. New York: W. W. Norton and Company.
Donald, M. (1991), *Origins of the Modern Mind: Three Stages in the Evolution of Culture and Cognition*. Cambridge, MA: Harvard University Press.
Donald, M. (2001), *A Mind So Rare: The Evolution of Human Consciousness*. New York: W. W. Norton and Company.
Downie, J. (2013a), *At the Limits of Art: A Literary Study of Aelius Aristides' Hieroi Logoi*. Oxford Scholarship Online. https://doi.org/10.1093/acprof:oso/9780199 924875.001.0001
Downie, J. (2013b), 'Dream hermeneutics in Aelius Aristides' Hieroi Logoi'. In: S. M. Oberhelman (ed.), *Dreams, Healing, and Medicine in Greece: From Antiquity to the Present*. Farnham: Ashgate, pp.109–128.
Du Bouchet, J., and Chandezon, C. (eds) (2012), *Études sur Artémidore et l'interprétation des rêves 1*. Nanterre: Presses Universitaires de Paris Ouest.
Dugas, M. J., Gosselin, P., and Ladouceur, R. (2001), 'Intolerance of uncertainty and worry: Investigating specificity in a nonclinical sample'. *Cognitive Therapy and Research* 25 (5), 551–558.
Dunn, A. J. (2005), 'Nervous and immune system interactions'. *eLS*. https://doi.org/10.1038/npg.els.0004068
Edelstein, L. (1943), *The Hippocratic Oath, Text, Translation and Interpretation*. Baltimore, MD: Johns Hopkins University Press.
Edelstein, E. J., and Edelstein, L. (1998 [1945]), *Asclepius: A Collection and Interpretation of the Testimonies*. 2 vols. Baltimore, MD: Johns Hopkins University Press.
Egnew, T. R. (2005), 'The meaning of healing: Transcending suffering'. *Annals of Family Medicine* 3 (3), 255–262.
Ehrhardt, N. (1989), 'Apollon Ietros. Ein verschollener Gott in Ionien?'. *Istanbuler Mitteilungen* 39, 115–122.
Eidinow, E. (2014), 'Oracles and oracle-sellers. An ancient market in futures'. In D. Engels and P. Van Nuffelen (eds), *Religion and Competition in Antiquity*. Brussels: Éditions Latomus, pp. 55–95.
Eippert, F., Bingel, U., Schoell, E. D., Yacubian, J., Klinger, R., Lorenz, J., and Büchel, C. (2009a), 'Activation of the opioidergic descending pain control system underlies placebo analgesia'. *Neuron* 63, 533–543.
Eippert, F., Finsterbusch, J., Bingel, U., and Büchel, C. (2009b), 'Direct evidence for spinal cord involvement in placebo analgesia'. *Science* 326, 404.

Eisenberg, L. (1977), 'The search of care'. *Daedalus* 106, 235–246.

Enck, P., Benedetti, F., and Schedlowski, M. (2008), 'New insights into the placebo and nocebo responses'. *Neuron* 59, 195–206.

Erickson, M. H., Rossi, E. L., and Rossi, S. I. (1976), *Hypnotic Realities: The Induction of Clinical Hypnosis and Forms of Indirect Suggestion*. New York: Irvington Publishers.

Fardo, F., Allen, M., Jegindø, E-M. E., Angrilli, A., and Roepstorff, A. (2015), 'Neurocognitive evidence for mental imagery-driven hypoalgesic and hyperalgesic pain regulation'. *NeuroImage* 120, 350–361.

Ferguson, E. (2003 [1987]), *Backgrounds of Early Christianity*. Grand Rapids, MI: W. B. Eerdmans.

Festugière, A. J. (1954), *Personal Religion Among the Greeks*. Berkeley, CA: University of California Press.

Finkler, K., and Correa, M. (1996), 'Factors influencing patient perceived recovery in Mexico'. *Social Science and Medicine* 42, 199–207.

Flanagan, O. J. (1997), 'Prospects for a unified theory of consciousness or, what dreams are made of'. In N. J. Block, O. J. Flanagan and G. Güzeldere (eds), *The Nature of Consciousness: Philosophical Debates*. (Bradford Books). Cambridge, MA: MIT Press, pp. 97–110.

Flaten, M. G., Simonsen, T., and Olsen, H. (1999), 'Drug-related information generates placebo and nocebo responses that modify the drug response'. *Psychosomatic Medicine* 61, 250–255.

Flower, M. A. (2008), *The Seer in Ancient Greece*. Berkeley, CA: University of California Press.

Fowler, H. N. (1921), *Plato in Twelve Volumes*, Vol. 12. Cambridge, MA: Harvard University Press; London: William Heinemann Ltd. 1921.

Freeston, M. H., Rhéaume, J., Letarte, H., Dugas, M. J., and Ladouceur, R. (1994), 'Why do people worry?'. *Personality and Individual Differences* 17, 791–802.

Frith, C. D., and Frith, U. (2012), 'Mechanisms of social cognition'. *Annual Review of Psychology* 63, 287–313.

Gallagher, E. J., Viscoli, C. M., and Horwitz, R. I. (1993), 'The relationship of treatment adherence to the risk of death after myocardial infarction in women'. *Journal of the American Medical Association* 270, 742–744.

Geertz, A. W. (1999), 'Definition as analytical strategy in the study of religion'. *Historical Reflections/Reflexions Historiques* 25 (3), 445–475.

Geertz, A. W. (2004), 'Cognitive approaches to the study of religion'. In P. Antes, A. W. Geertz and R. R. Warne (eds), *New Approaches to the Study of Religion: Textual, Comparative, Sociological, and Cognitive Approaches*. Berlin: W. De Gruyter, pp. 347–400.

Geertz, A. W. (2010), 'Brain, body and culture: A biocultural theory of religion'. *Method and Theory in the Study of Religion* 22 (4), 304–321.

Geertz, A. W. (2016), 'Cognitive science'. In M. Stausberg and S. Engler (eds), *The*

Oxford Handbook of the Study of Religion. Oxford: Oxford University Press, 97–111.

Geertz, A. W. (2020), 'How did ignorance become fact in American religious studies? A reluctant reply to Ivan Strenski'. *SMSR - Studi e Materiali di Storia delle Religioni* 86 (1), 365–403.

Geertz, C. (1990), *The Interpretation of Cultures: Selected Essays*. New York: Basic Books.

Gehrke, J. (2003), *History of the Hellenistic World* (in Greek). Translated by A. Chaniotis. Athens: MIET.

Gelbman, F. (1967), 'The physician, the placebo and the placebo effect'. *Ohio State Medical Journal* 63, 1459–1461.

Georgoulaki, E. (1997), 'Votives in the shape of human body parts: Shaping a framework'. *Platon* 49, 188–206.

Gesler, M. W. (1992), 'Therapeutic landscapes: Medical issues in light of the new cultural geography'. *Social Science and Medicine* 34, 735–746.

Gesler, M. W. (1993), 'Therapeutic landscapes: Theory and a case study of Epidaurus, Greece'. *Environment and Planning D: Society and Space* 11 (2), 171–189.

Gesler, M. W. (1996), 'Lourdes: Healing in a place of pilgrimage'. *Health and Place* 2, 95–105.

Gesler, M. W. (1998), 'Bath's reputation as a healing place'. In R. Kearns and W. Gesler (eds), *Putting Health into Place. Landscape, Identity, and Well-being*. Syracuse, NY: Syracuse University Press, pp. 17–35.

Gesler, M. W. (2003), *Healing Places*. New York: Rowman and Littlefield.

Ginouvès, R. (1959), *L'Etablissement thermal de Gortys d'Arcadie*. Paris: J. Vrin.

Ginouvès, R. (1962), *Balaneutiké: Recherches sur le bain dans l'antiquité grecque*. (Bibliothèque des écoles françaises d'Athènes et de Rome 200). Paris: E. de Boccard.

Girard, P. (1831), *L'Asclépieion d'Athènes d'après de récentes décou- vertes*. Paris: E. Thorin.

Glenberg, A. M., Schroeder, J. L., and Robertson, D. A. (1998), 'Averting the gaze disengages the environment and facilitates remembering'. *Memory and Cognition* 26 (4), 651–658.

Glicksohn, J. (1991), 'The induction of an altered state of consciousness as a function of sensory environment and experience seeking'. *Personality and Individual Differences* 12 (10), 1057–1066.

Glinister, F. (2007), 'Reconsidering religious romanization'. In C. E. Schultz and P. B. Harvey (eds), *Religion in Republican Italy*. Cambridge: Cambridge University Press, pp. 10–32.

Goebel, M. U., Hubell, D., Kou, W., Janssen, O. E., Katsarava, Z., Limmroth, V., and Schedlowski, M. (2005), 'Behavioral conditioning with interferon beta-1a in humans'. *Physiology and Behavior* 84, 807–814.

Goebel, M. U., Meykadeh, N., Kou, W., Schedlowski, M., and Hengge, U. R. (2009),

'Behavioral conditioning of antihistamine effects in patients with allergic rhinitis'. *Psychother Psychosom* 77, 227–234.

Goebel, M. U., Trebst, A. E., Steiner, J., Xie, Y. F, Exton, M. S., Frede, S., Canbay, A. E., Michel, M. C., Heemann, U., and Schedlowski, M. (2002), 'Behavioral conditioning of immunosuppression is possible in humans'. *FASEB Journal* 16, 1869–1873.

Goetz, C. G., J. Wuu, M. P. McDermott, C. H. Adler, S. Fahn, C. R. Freed, R. A. Hauser, W. C. Olanow, I. Shoulson, P. K. Tandon, and S. Leurgans (2008), 'Placebo response in Parkinson's disease: Comparisons among 11 trials covering medical and surgical interventions'. *Movement Disorders* 23 (5), 690–699.

Gordon, R. (1995), 'The healing event in Graeco-Roman folk-medicine'. In P. J. van Der Eijk, H. F. J. Horstmanshoff and P. H. Schrijvers (eds), *Ancient Medicine in Its Socio-Cultural Context: Papers Read at the Congress Held at Leiden University 13-15 April 1992*, Vol. II, Amsterdam, Atlant: Rodopi, pp. 363–376.

Gordon, R., and Reynolds, J. (2003), 'Roman inscriptions 1995–2000'. *Journal of Roman Studies* 93, 212–294.

Gorrini, M. (2001), 'Gli eroi salutari dell'Attica'. *ASAtene* 79, 299–315.

Gorrini, M. (2005), 'The Hippocratic impact on healing cults: The archaeological evidence in Attica'. In P. J. van der Eijk (ed.), *Hippocrates in Context.* Leiden: Brill, pp. 135–156.

Gotzsche, P. C. (1994), 'Is there logic in the placebo?' *Lancet* 344, 925–926.

Gracely, R. H., Dubner, R., Deeter, W. R., and Wolskee, P. J. (1985), ''Clinicians' expectations influence placebo analgesia [Letter]'. *Lancet* 1, 43.

Graf, F. (2009), *Apollo.* (Gods and Heroes of the Ancient World). New York: Routledge.

Graham, L. R. (1994), 'Dialogic dreams: Creative selves coming into life in the flow of time'. *American Ethnologist* 21 (4), 723–745.

Green, P. (1990), *Alexander to Actium. The Hellenistic Age.* London: Thames and Hudson.

Greenfield, S. (2000), *The Private Life of the Brain.* Harmondsworth: Penguin.

Greenhill, W. A. (1867), 'Aegle (5)'. In W. Smith (ed.), *Dictionary of Greek and Roman Biography and Mythology 1.* Boston, MA: Little, Brown and Co.

Griffith, A. B. (2014), 'Dead religion, live minds: Memory and recall of the mithraic bull-slaying scene'. *Journal of Cognitive Historiography* 1 (1), 72–89.

Griffith, G. T. (1935), *The Mercenaries of the Hellenistic World.* Cambridge: Cambridge University Press.

Grmek, Mirko D. (1989), *Diseases in the ancient Greek world.* Translated by M. Muellner and. D. L. Muellner. Baltimore, MD: Johns Hopkins University Press.

Grünbaum, A. (1981), 'The placebo concept'. *Behavior Research and Therapy* 19, 157–167.

Guthrie, S. (1992), *Faces in the Clouds: A New Theory of Religion.* New York: Oxford University Press.

Habicht, C. (1969), *Altertümer von Pergamon. Band Viii. 3: Die Inschriften des Asclepeios.*

Berlin: W. De Gruyter.

Habicht, C. (1985), *Pausanias' Guide to Ancient Greece*. Berkeley, CA: University of California Press.

Hamilton, M. (1906), *Incubation or The Cure of Disease in Pagan Temple and Christian Churches*. St. Andrews, Scotland: W. C. Henderson and Sons.

Hamilton, R. (2000), *Treasure Map. A Guide to the Delian Inventories*. Ann Arbor, MI: University of Michigan Press.

Hampton, J. A. (1997), 'Conceptual combination'. In K. Lamberts and D. Shanks (eds), *Knowledge, Concepts, and Categories*. (Studies in Cognition). Cambridge, MA: The MIT Press, pp. 133–159.

Hankinson, R. J. (1998a), 'Magic, religion and science: Divine and human in the Hippocratic Corpus'. *Apeiron* 31, 1–34.

Hankinson, R. J. (1998b), *Cause and Explanation in Ancient Greek Thought*. Oxford: Clarendon Press.

Harper, K. (2017), *The Fate of Rome: Climate, Disease, and the End of an Empire*. Princeton, NJ: Princeton University Press.

Harris, W. V. (2009), *Dreams and Experience in Classical Antiquity*. Cambridge, MA: Harvard University Press.

Harris, W. V., and Holmes, B. (eds) (2008), *Aelius Aristides between Greece, Rome, and the Gods*. (Columbia Studies in the Classical Tradition). Leiden: Brill.

Harris-McCoy, D. E. (2012), *Artemidorus' Oneirocritica: Text, Translation, and Commentary*. Oxford: Oxford University Press.

Harrisson, J. (2013), *Dreams and Dreaming in the Roman Empire: Cultural Memory and Imagination*. London: Bloomsbury Academic.

Harrisson, J. (2014), 'The development of the practice of incubation in the ancient world'. In D. Michaelides (ed.), *Medicine and Healing in the Ancient Mediterranean World*. Oxford: Oxbow Books, pp. 284–290.

Hart, D. G. (1966), 'Ancient coins and medicine'. *Canadian Medical Association Journal* 94, 77–89.

Hart, D. G. (2000), *Asclepius, the God of Medicine*. London: Royal Society of Medicine Press.

Hartig, T., Evans, G. W., Jamner, L. D., Davis, D. S., and Gärling, T. (2003), 'Tracking restoration in natural and urban field settings'. *Journal of Environmental Psychology* 23, 109–123.

Hartmann, E. (1998), *Dreams and Nightmares: The New Theory on the Origin and Meaning of Dreams*. New York: Plenum Press.

Hatfield, G., and Pittman, H. (2013), *Evolution of Mind, Brain, and Culture*. Philadelphia, PA: University of Pennsylvania Press.

Hayes, P. (1979), 'The naïve physics manifesto'. In D. Michie (ed.), *Expert Systems in the Micro-electronic Age*. Edinburgh: Edinburgh University Press, pp. 242–270.

Heerwagen, J. (1990), 'The psychological aspects of windows and window design'.

In K. H. Anthony, J. Choi and B. Orland (eds), *Proceedings of the 21st Annual Conference of the Environmental Design Research Association.* Oklahoma City, OK: EDRA, pp. 269–280.

Hemingway, B. (2008), *The Dream in Classical Greece: Debates and Practices.* PhD dissertation. Trinity: The Queen's College.

Henrich, J. (2015), *The Secret of Our Success: How Culture is Driving Human Evolution, Domesticating Our Species, and Making Us Smarter.* Princeton, NJ: Princeton University Press.

Henrichs, A. (2010), 'What is a Greek god'. In J. Bremmer and A. Erskine (eds), *The Gods of Ancient Greece: Identities and Transformations.* Edinburgh: Edinburgh University Press, pp. 19–39.

Herrnstein, R. J. (1962), 'Placebo effect in the rat'. *Science* 138, 677–678.

Herzog, R. (1928), *Heilige Gesetze von Kos.* Berlin: Verlag der Akademie der Wissenschaften, in Kommission bei de Gruyter.

Herzog, R. (1931), *Die Wunderheilungen von Epidauros.* Leipzig: Dieterich.

Heyes, C., and Dickinson, A. (1990), 'The intentionality of animal action'. *Mind and Language* 5 (1), 87–103. https://doi.org/10.1111/j.1468-0017.1990.tb00154.x

Hobson, A. J. (1988), *The Dreaming Brain.* New York: Basic Books.

Hobson, A. J. (1994), *The Chemistry of Consciousness: How the Brain Changes its Mind.* New York: Little, Brown.

Hobson, A. J., and Stickgold, R. (1994), 'Dreaming: A neurocognitive approach'. *Consciousness and Cognition* 3 (1), 1–15.

Hobson, A. J., Pace-Schott, E. F., and Stickgold, R. (2000), 'Dreaming and the brain: Toward a cognitive neuroscience of conscious states'. *Behavioral and Brain Sciences* 23 (6), 793–1121.

Hoffmann, A. (1998), 'The Roman remodeling of the Asklepieion'. In H. Koester (ed.), *Pergamon, Citadel of the Gods: Archaeological Record, Literary Description, and Religious Development.* (Harvard Theological Studies 46). Harrisburg, PA: Trinity Press International, pp. 41–61.

Hofmann, B. (2002), 'On the triad disease, illness and sickness'. *Journal of Medicine and Philosophy* 27 (6), 651–673.

Hofmann, B. (2017), 'Disease, illness, and sickness'. In M. Solomon, J. E. Simon and H. Kincaid (eds), *The Routledge Companion to Philosophy of Medicine.* (Routledge Philosophy Companions). New York: Routledge, pp. 16–26.

Holmes, B. (2008), 'Aelius Aristides' illegible body'. In W. V. Harris and B. Holmes (ed.), *Aelius Aristides: Between Greece, Rome and the Gods.* Leiden: Brill, pp. 81–114.

Holowchak, A. M. (2001), 'Interpreting dreams for corrective regimen: Diagnostic dreams in Greco-Roman medicine'. *Journal of the History of Medicine and Allied Sciences* 56 (4), 382–399. https://doi.org/10.1093/jhmas/56.4.382.

Holowchak, A. M. (2002), *Ancient science and dreams. Oneirology in Graeco-Roman*

Antiquity. New York: University Press of America.
Horstmanshoff, H. F. J (2004a), 'Asclepius and temple medicine in Aelius Aristides' *Sacred Tales*'. In H. F. J. Horstmanshoff and M. Stol (eds), *Magic and Rationality in Ancient Near Eastern and Graeco-Roman Medicine*. (Studies in Ancient Medicine 27). Leiden: Brill, pp. 325-342.
Horstmanshoff, H. F. J (2004b), 'Aelius Aristides: A suitable case for treatment'. In B. Borg (ed.), *Paideia: The World of the Second Sophistic*. (Millennium Studies 27). New York: W. De Gruyter, pp. 277-292.
Horwitz, R. I., and Horwitz, S. M. (1993), 'Adherence to treatment and health outcomes'. *Archives of Internal Medicine* 153, 1863-1868.
Howard, P. (2006), *The Owner's Manual for the Brain - Everyday Applications from Mind-Brain Research*. Austin, TX: Bard Press.
Hucklebridge, F. (2002), 'Behavioral conditioning of the immune systems'. *International Review of Neurobiology* 52, 325-351.
Hughes, J. (2008), 'Fragmentation as metaphor in the Classical healing sanctuary'. *Social History of Medicine* 21 (2), 217-236. https://doi.org/10.1093/shm/hkn 034.
Hulskamp, M. (2013), 'The value of dream diagnosis in the medical praxis of the Hippocratics and Galen'. In S. M. Oberhelman (ed.), *Dreams, Healing, and Medicine in Greece: From Antiquity to the Present*. Farnham: Ashgate, pp. 33-68.
Humphrey, N. (1995), *Leaps of Faith Science, Miracles, and the Search for Supernatural Consolation*. New York: Basic Books.
Humphrey, N. (2002), *The Mind Made Flesh: Essays from the Frontiers of Psychology and Evolution*. Oxford: Oxford University Press.
Humphrey, N. (2005) 'Placebo effect'. Manuscript provided by author (published version is available in R. Gregory (ed.), *Oxford Companion to the Mind*, 2nd edition, Oxford: Oxford University Press, 2004).
Humphreys, G. W., and Forde, E. M. E. (2001), 'Hierarchies, similarity, and interactivity in object recognition: "Categoryspecific" neuropsychological deficits'. *Behavioral and Brain Sciences* 24, 453-509.
Hutchins, E. (1995), *Cognition in the Wild*. Cambridge, MA: MIT Press.
Hutchins, E. (2010), 'Cognitive Ecology'. *Topics in Cognitive Science* 2, 705-715.
Hyland, M. E., Whalley, B., and Geraghty, A. W. A. (2007), 'Dispositional predictors of placebo responding: A motivational interpretation of flower essence and gratitude therapy'. *Journal of Psychosomatic Research* 62, 331-340.
Hyman, I. E., Husband, T. H., and Billings, F. J. (1995), 'False memories of childhood experiences'. *Applied Cognitive Psychology* 9, 181-197.
Iacoboni, M. (2009), 'Imitation, empathy, and mirror neurons'. *Annual Review of Psychology* 60, 653-670.
Illich, I. (1976), *Limits to Medicine*. London: Marion Boyars.
Irving, L. M., Snyder, C. R., and Crowson, J. J. (1998), 'Hope and coping with cancer

by college women'. *Journal of Personality* 66 (2), 195-214.

Irwin, M., and K. Vedhara (2005), *Human Psychoneuroimmunology*. Oxford: Oxford University Press.

Israelowich, I. (2012), *Society, Medicine and Religion in the Sacred Tales of Aelius Aristides*. Leiden, Boston: Brill.

Israelowich, I. (2014), 'Physicians as figures of authority in the Roman courts and the attitude towards mental diseases in the Roman courts during the High Empire'. *Historia* 63 (4), 445-462.

Israelowich, I. (2015), *Patients and Healers in the High Roman Empire*. Baltimore, MD: Johns Hopkins University Press.

Jensen, J. S. (2010), 'Doing it the other way round: Religion as a basic case of "Normative Cognition"'. *Method and Theory in the Study of Religion* 22 (4), 322-329.

Jensen, J. S. (2013), 'Normative cognition in culture and religion'. *Journal for the Cognitive Science of Religion* 1 (1), 47-70. https://doi.org/10.1558/jcsr.v1i1.47

Jensen, J. S. (2016), 'How institutions work in shared intentionality and "we-mode" social cognition'. *Topoi* 35, 301-312. https://doi.org/10.1007/s11245-015-9306-7

Johnson, M. (1993), *Moral Imagination. Implications of cognitive science for ethics*. Chicago, IL: University of Chicago Press.

Johnson, M. K. (2001), 'Psychology of false memories'. In N. J. Smelser and P. B. Baltes (eds), *International Encyclopedia of the Social and Behavioral Sciences*. New York: Pergamon, pp. 5254-5259.

Johnson, M. K., and Raye, C. L. (1998), 'False memories and confabulation'. *Trends in Cognitive Sciences* 2 (4), 137-145.

Johnston, S. I. (2008), *Ancient Greek Divination*. Oxford: Wiley-Blackwell.

Jonas, W. B., and Chez, R. A. (2004), 'Toward optimal healing environments in health care'. *The Journal of Alternative and Complementary Medicine* 10 (Suppl. 1), S1-S6. https://doi.org/10.1089/acm.2004.10.S-1.

Jonas, W. B., and Chez, R. A. (2006), 'Implementing and evaluating optimal healing environments'. In D. Rakel and N. Faass (eds), *Complementary Medicine in Clinical Practice: Integrative Practice in American Healthcare*. Sudbury, MA: Jones and Barlett, pp. 517-522.

Jones, C. (1998), 'Aelius Aristides and the Asklepieion'. In H. Koester (ed.), *Pergamon, Citadel of the Gods: Archaeological Record, Literary Description, and Religious Development*. (Harvard Theological Studies 46). Harrisburg, PA: Trinity Press International, pp. 63-76.

Jones, D. W. (1999), *Peak Sanctuaries and Sacred Caves in Minoan Crete: Comparison of Artifacts*. Jonsered, Sweden: Åström.

Jones, W.H.S. (ed. and trans.) (1868), *Hippocrates Collected Works I*. Cambridge: Harvard University Press. 1868.

Jones, W.H.S. (trans) (1923) *Hippocrates. Prognostic. Regimen in Acute Diseases. The*

Sacred Disease. The Art. Breaths. Law. Decorum. Physician (Ch. 1). Dentition. Cambridge, MA: Harvard University Press.
Jones, H. L. (trans.) (1924), *The Geography of Strabo.* Cambridge, MA: Harvard University Press.
Jones, W. H. S., and Ormerod, H. A. (trans.) (1918), *Pausanias: Description of Greece.* 4 volumes. Cambridge, MA: Harvard University Press.
Jopling, D. (2008), *Talking Cures and Placebo Effects.* Oxford: Oxford University Press.
Jost, M. (1992), *Aspects de la vie religieuse en Grèce. Du début du Ve siècle à la fin du IIIe siècle av. J.-C.* Paris: Sedes.
Jouanna, J. (1999), *Hippocrates.* Translated by M. B. DeBevoise. Baltimore, MD: Johns Hopkins University Press.
Jouanna, J. (2003) (ed. and trans.), *Hippocrate: Oeuvres,* vol. 2, part 3: *La maladie sacrée.* Paris: Les Belles Lettres, 130-131.
Jouanna, J. (2012), *Greek Medicine from Hippocrates to Galen: Selected Papers.* (Studies in ancient medicine 40). Translated by N. Allies; edited with a preface by P. van der Eijk. Leiden: Brill.
Jowett, B. (trans.) (1956), *Plato's Symposium.* New York : Liberal Arts Press.
Kahn, D., Krippner, S., and Combs, A. (2000), 'Dreaming and the self-organizing brain'. *Journal of Consciousness Studies* 7 (7), 4-11.
Kaplan, S. H., Greenfield, S., and Ware, J. E. (1989), 'Assessing the effects of physician-patient interactions on the outcomes of chronic disease'. *Medical Care* 27, 110-127.
Kaptchuk, T. J. (2002), 'The placebo effect in alternative medicine: Can the performance of a healing ritual have clinical significance?'. *Annals of Internal Medicine* 136, 817-825.
Kaptchuk, T. J., and Eisenberg, D. M. (1998), 'The persuasive appeal of alternative medicine'. *Annals of Internal Medicine* 129 (12), 1061-1065.
Kaptchuk, T. J., Friedlander, E., Kelley, J. M., Sanchez, M. N., Kokkotou, E., Singer, J. P., Kowalczykowski, M., Miller, F. G, Kirsch, I., and Lembo, A. J. (2010), 'Placebos without deception: A randomized controlled trial in irritable bowel syndrome'. *PLoS ONE* 5 (12). Retrieved from www.plosone.org/article/info%3Adoi%2F10.1371%2Fjournal.pone.0015591 (accessed 16 September 2013). https://doi.org/10.1371/journal.pone.0015591.
Kaptchuk, T. J., Kelley, J. M., Deykin, A., Wayne, P. M., Lasagna, L. C., Epstein, I. O., Kirsch, I., and Wechsler, M. E. (2008), 'Do "placebo responders" exist?'. *Contemporary Clinical Trials* 29 (4), 587-595.
Kaptchuk, T. J., Miller, F. G., and Colloca, L. (2009), 'The placebo effect illness and interpersonal healing'. *Perspectives in Biology and Medicine* 52 (4), 518-539.
Kapur, S. (2003), 'Psychosis as a state of aberrant salience: A framework linking biology, phenomenology, and pharmacology in schizophrenia'. *American Journal of Psychiatry* 160, 13-23.
Kastriotis, P. (1918), 'Triccas' Asclepeion' (in Greek). *Archaeological Newspaper,*

65–67.

Kearns, E. (1989), *The Heroes of Attica*. London: Institute of Classical Studies.

Kee, H. (1983), *Miracle in the Early Christian World: A Study in Sociohistorical Method*. New Haven, CT: Yale University Press.

Kemeny, M. E., Rosenwasser, L. J., Panettieri, R. A., Rose, R. M., Berg-Smith, S. M., and Kline, J. N. (2007), 'Placebo response in asthma: A robust and objective phenomenon'. *Journal of Allergy and Clinical Immunology* 119 (6), 1375–1381.

Kennedy, J. S. (1992), *The New Anthropomorphism*. Cambridge: Cambridge University Press.

Kerényi, K. (1945), 'Heros Iatros'. *Eranos Jahrbuch* 12, 33–54.

Kerényi, K. (1959), *Asclepios: Archetypical Image of the Physician's Existence*. Translated by Ralph Manheim. Princeton, NJ: Princeton University Press.

Khachatiurians, A. K. (2006), 'Therapeutic landscapes: A critical analysis'. Master's thesis, Simon Fraser University, Stoke-on-Trent.

Kienle, G. S, and Kiene, H. (1996), 'Placebo effect and placebo concept: A critical methodological and conceptual analysis of reports on the magnitude of the placebo effect'. *Alternative Therapies In Health And Medicine* 2, 39–54.

Kindt, J. (2012), *Rethinking Greek Religion*. Cambridge: Cambridge University Presss.

Kirmayer, L. J. (1993), 'Healing and the invention of metaphor: The effectiveness of symbols revisited'. *Culture, Medicine and Psychiatry* 17, 161–195.

Klauer, K., and Musch, C. (2003), 'Affective priming: Findings and theories'. In J. Musch and K. C. Klauer (eds), *The Psychology of Evaluation: Affective Processes in Cognition and Emotion*. Mahwah, NJ: Psychology Press, pp. 7–49.

Kleijwegt, M. (1994) 'Beans, baths and the barber … a sacred law from Thuburbos Maius'. *Antiquités Africaines* 30, 209–220.

Kleinman, A. (1980), *Patients and Healers in the Context of Culture: An Exploration of the Borderland Between Anthropology, Medicine, and Psychiatry*. Berkeley, CA: University of California Press.

Kleinman, A. (1988), *The Illness Narratives: Suffering, Healing, and the Human Condition*. New York: Basic Books.

Kleisiaris, C. F, Sfakianakis, C., and Papathanasiou, I. V. (2014), 'Health care practices in ancient Greece: The Hippocratic ideal'. *Journal of Medical Ethics and History of Medicine* 7 (6).

Kline, A. S. (trans.) (2014), *Ovid's Metamorphoses*. London: CreateSpace Independent Publishing Platform.

Klinger, R., Soost, S., Flor, H., and Worm M. (2007), 'Classical conditioning and expectancy in placebo hypoalgesia: A randomized controlled study in patients with atopic dermatitis and persons with healthy skin'. *Pain* 128, 31–39.

Klostergaard Petersen, A. (2009), 'Alexandrian Judaism: Rethinking a problematical cultural category'. In G. Hinge, and J. Krasilnikoff (eds), *Alexandria. A Cultural and Religious Melting Pot*. Aarhus: Aarhus University Press, pp. 115–143.

Kluger, M. J., Kozak, W., Conn, C. A. Leon, L. R., and Soszynski, D. (1996), 'The adaptive value of fever'. *Infectious Disease Clinics of North America* 10, 1–20.

Knox, A. D. (ed. and trans.) (1922), *Herodas: The Mimes and Fragments*. Cambridge: Cambridge University Press.

Kranz, P. (2010), *Hygieia: Die Frau an Asklepios' Seite: Untersuchungen zu Darstellung und Funktion in klassischer und hellenistischer Zeit unter Einbeziehung der Gestalt des Asklepios*. Möhnesee: Bibliopolis.

Krippner, S., and Combs, A. (2000), 'Self-organization in the dreaming brain'. *Journal of Mind and Behavior* 21, 399–412.

Krostenko, B. (2000), 'Beyond (dis)belief: Rhetorical form and religious symbol in Cicero's *de divinatione*'. *Transactions of the American Philological Association* 130, 353–391.

Laland, K. N. (2017), *Darwin's Unfinished Symphony: How Culture Made the Human Mind*. Princeton, NJ: Princeton University Press.

Lang, M. (1977), *Cure and Cult in Ancient Corinth: A Guide to the Asclepeio*. Princeton, NJ: American School of Classical Studies at Athens.

Lasagna, L., Mosteller, F., Von Felsinger, J. M., and Beecher, H. K. (1954), 'A study of the placebo response'. *American Journal of Medicine* 16 (6), 770–779.

Laskaris, J. (1999), 'Archaic healing cults as a source for Hippocratic pharmacology'. In I. Garofalo, A. Lami, D. Manetti and A. Roselli (eds), *Aspetti della terapia nel Corpus Hippocraticum: Atti del atti del IXe Colloque International Hippocratique, Pisa, 25–29 Settembre 1996*. (Studi/Accademia toscana di scienze e lettere 'La colombaria' 183). Florence: L. S. Olschki, pp. 1–12.

Laskaris, J. (2002), *The Art is Long. On the Sacred Disease and the Scientific Tradition*. Leiden: Brill.

Laumann, K., Gärling, T., and Stormark, K. M. (2003), 'Selective attention and heart rate responses to natural and urban environments'. *Journal of Environmental Psychology* 23, 125–134.

Lawson, E. T., and McCauley, R. N. (1990), *Rethinking Religion: Connecting Cognition and Culture*. Cambridge: Cambridge University Press.

Lefantzis, M., and Jensen, J. T. (2009), 'The Athenian asklepieion on the south slope of the Akropolis: Early development, ca. 420–360 B.C'. In J. T. Jensen, G. Hinge, P. Schultz and B. Wickkiser (eds), *Aspects of Ancient Greek Cult Context, Ritual and Iconography*. (Aarhus Studies in Mediterranean Antiquity VIII). Aarhus: Aarhus University Press, pp. 91–124.

Leuchter, A. F., Cook, I. A., Witte, E. A., Morgan, M. et al. (2002), 'Changes in brain function of depressed subjects during treatment with placebo'. *American Journal of Psychiatry* 159, 122–129.

Leuci, V. A. (1993), 'Dream-technical terms in the Greco-Roman world'. PhD dissertation, University of Missouri, Columbia, MO.

Leventhal, H., Nerenz, D., and Strauss, A. (1982), 'Self-regulation and the mechanisms for symptom appraisal'. In D. Mechanic (ed.), *Psychosocial Epidemiology*.

(Symptoms, Illness Behavior, and Help 3). New York: Neale Watson, pp. 55–86.
Leventi, I. (2003), *Hygieia in Classical Greek Art*. (Archaiognosia Suppl. 2). Athens: Kardamitsa.
Liberman, R. P. (1967), 'The elusive placebo reactor'. *Neuropsychopharmacology* 5, 557–566.
Lichko, A. E. (1959), 'Conditioned reflex hypoglycemia in man'. *Pavlov Journal of Higher Nervous Activity* 9, 731–737.
LiDonnici, L. R. (1992), 'Compositional background of the Epidaurian iamata'. *American Journal of Philology* 113, 25–41.
LiDonnici, L. R. (1995), *The Epidaurian Inscriptions: Text, Translation, and Commentary*. Atlanta, Georgia: Scholars Press.
Lin, A., Adolphs, R., and Rangel, A. (2012), 'Social and monetary reward learning engage overlapping neural substrates'. *Social Cognitive and Affective Neuroscience* 7 (3), 274–281.
Lincoln, B. (1989), *Discourse and the Construction of Society: Comparative Studies of Myth, Ritual, and Classification*. New York: Oxford University Press.
Linderski, J. (1982), 'Cicero and Roman divination'. *La Parola del Passato* 37, 12–38.
Lioulias, S. (2010), 'The worship of Asclepius in Macedonia'. Master's thesis, Aristotle University of Thessaloniki, Thessaloniki, Greece.
Lloyd, G. E. R. (1979), *Magic, Reason and Experience*. Cambridge: Cambridge University Press.
Lloyd, G. E. R. (1983), *Science, Folklore and Ideology: Studies in the Life Sciences in Ancient Greece*. Cambridge, MA: Hackett Publishing Company.
Lloyd, G. E. R. (1987), *The Revolutions of Wisdom*. Berkeley, CA: University of California Press.
Lloyd, G. E. R. (2003), *In the Grip of Disease*. Oxford: Oxford University Press.
Loftus, E. F. (1997), 'Creating false memories'. *Scientific American* 277 (3), 70–75.
Loftus, E. F., and Pickrell, J. E. (1995), 'The formation of false memories'. *Psychiatric Annals* 25, 720–725.
Lohr, V. I., and Pearson-Mims, C. H. (2006), 'Responses to scenes with spreading, rounded, and conical tree forms'. *Environment and Behavior* 38, 667–688.
Longrigg, J. (1993), *Greek Rational Medicine: Philosophy and Medicine from Alcmaeon to the Alexandrians*. New York: Routledge.
Longrigg, J. (1998), *Greek Medicine from the Heroic to the Hellenistic Age: A Source Book*. London: Duckworth.
Lui, F., Colloca L., Duzzi D., Anchisi, D. et al. (2010), 'Neural bases of conditioned placebo analgesia'. *Pain* 151, 815–823.
Lundhaug, H. (2014), 'Memory and early monastic literary practices: A cognitive perspective'. *Journal of Cognitive Historiography* 1 (1), 98–120.
Lyttkens, C. H. (2011), 'Health, economics and ancient Greek medicine'. *The Journal of Economic Asymmetries* 8, 165–192.

MacMullen, R. (1976), *Roman Government's Response to Crisis, A.D. 235-337*. New Haven, CT: Yale University Press.
Malafouris, L. (2010), 'The brain-artefact interface (BAI): A challenge for archaeology and cultural neuroscience'. *Social Cognitive and Affective Neuroscience* 5 (2-3), 264-273.
Mann J. (trans.) (2012), *Hippocrates: On the Art of Medicine*. Leiden: Brill.
Marler, P., and Ristau, C. A. (eds) (1990), *Cognitive Ethology: Essays in Honor of Donald R. Griffin*. (Comparative Cognition and Neuroscience Series). New York: Psychology Press.
Marshall, H. F. (1909), 'Some recent acquisitions of the British Museum'. *Journal of Hellenic Studies* 19, 151-167.
Martin, A. (2001), 'Functional neuroimaging of semantic memory'. In R. Cabeza and A. Kingstone (eds), *Handbook of functional neuroimaging of cognition. Cognitive Neuroscience*. Cambridge, MA: MIT Press, pp. 153-186.
Martin, L. H. (1994) 'The anti-individualistic ideology of Hellenistic culture'. *Numen* XLI (2), 117-140.
Martin, L. H. (2004), *Religions of the Hellesnistic Era* (in Greek). Translated by D. Xygalatas. Thessaloniki: Vanias.
Martin, L. H. (2012), 'Cognition and religion'. *Culture and Research*. 1, 25-42.
Martin, R., and Metzger, H. (1940-1941), 'Gortys [Arcadie]'. *Chronique des Fouilles et. Découvertes Archéologiques en Grèce en 1940 et 1941, Bulletin de correspondance hellénique* 64-65, 280-286.
Martin, R., and Metzger, H. (1942-1943), 'Gortys d'Arcadie'. *Chronique des Fouilles et Découvertes Archéologiques en Grèce en 1942. Bulletin de correspondance hellénique* 66-67, 334-336.
Martin, R., and Metzger, H. (1949), 'Recherches d'architecture et de topographie à l'Asclépiéion d'Athènes'. *Bulletin de correspondance hellénique* 73, 316-350.
Martin, R., and Metzger, H. (1992), *The Religion of the Ancient Greeks* (in Greek). Translated by A. Kardmitsa. Athens: Kardamitsa.
Martzavou, P. (2012), 'Dream, narrative, and the construction of hope in the "healing miracles" of Epidaurus'. In A. Chaniotis (ed.), *Unveiling Emotions: Sources and Methods for the Study of Emotions in the Greek World*. (Heidelberger Althistorische Beitrage und Epigraphische Studien 52). Stuttgart: Steiner Verlag.
Mattern, S. P. (2013), *The Prince of Medicine: Galen in the Roman Empire*. Oxford: Oxford University Press.
Mattocks, K. M., and Horwitz, R.I. (2000), 'Placebos, active control groups, and the unpredictability paradox'. *Biological Psychiatry* 47, 693-698.
Mayberg, H. S., Silva, J. A., Brannan, S. K., Tekell, J. L., Mahurin, R. K., McGinnis, S., and Jerabek, P. A. (2002), 'The functional neuroanatomy of the placebo'. *American Journal of Psychiatry* 159 (5), 728-737.
Mazzoni, G., Foan, L., Hyland, M. E., and Kirsch, I. (2010), 'The effects of observation

and gender on psychogenic symptoms'. *Health Psychology* 29, 181–185.

McCauley, R. N., and Lawson, E.T. (2002), *Bringing Ritual to Mind. Psychological Foundations of Cultural Forms*. Cambridge: Cambridge University Press.

McDonagh, B. (1989), *Turkey: The Aegean and Mediterranean Coasts*. London: A. & C. Black.

McKay, R., Efferson, C., Whitehouse, H., and Fehr, E. (2010), 'Wrath of god: Religious primes and punishment'. *Proceedings of the Royal Society B* 278 (1713), 1858–1863. https://doi.org/10.1098/rspb.2010.2125

McKechnie, P. (2014), *Outsiders in the Greek Cities in the Fourth Century BC*. London: Routledge Revivals.

McNair, D. M., Gardos, G., Haskell, D. S., and Fisher, S. (1979), 'Placebo response, placebo effect and two attributes'. *Psychopharmacology* 63 (3), 245–250.

McNamara, L. (2003–2004), 'Conjurers, purifiers, vagabonds and quacks? The clinical roles of the folk and Hippocratic healers of Classical Greece'. *Journal of the Classical Association of Victoria* 16–17, 2–25.

McPherson, K., Britton, A. R., and Wennberg, J. E. (1997), 'Are randomized controlled trials controlled? Patient preferences and unblind trials'. *Journal of the Royal Society of Medicine* 90 (12), 652–656.

Medvedev, V., Zavyalova, E. K., Ovchinnikov, B. V., and Posokhova, S. T. (1984), 'Functional structure of the placebo response'. *Fiziologiya Cheloveka* 10, 458–464.

Meier, C. A. (1967), *Ancient Incubation and Modern Psychotherapy*. Translated by M. Curtis. Evanston, IL: Northwestern University Press.

Melfi, M. (2007), *Il santuario di Asclepio a Lebena*. Athens: Scuola archeologica italiana di Atene.

Melfi, M. (2009), ' Lost sculptures from the Asklepieion of Lebena'. *Creta Antica* 11, 607–618.

Melfi, M. (2010), 'Rebuilding the myth of Asklepios at the sanctuary of Epidaurus in the Roman period'. In A. D. Rizakis and C. E. Lepenioti (eds), *Roman Peloponnese III. Society, Economy and Culture under the Roman Empire: Continuity and Innovation*. (Meletemata 63). Athens: National Hellenic Research Foundation, pp. 329–340.

Melfi, M. (2016), 'The archaeology of the asclepieum of Pergamum'. In D. A. Russell, M. Trapp and H.-G. Nesselrath (eds), *In Praise of Asclepius. Aelius Aristides, Selected Prose Hymns*. Tübingen: Mohr Siebeck, pp. 89–114.

Michenaud, G., and Dierkens, J. (1972), *Les reves dans les "Discours Sacres" d'Aelius Aristides*. Mons: University of Mons Press.

Mikalson, J. D. (2010), *Ancient Greek Religion*. Chichester: Wiley-Blackwell.

Miller, P. C. (1998), *Dreams in Late Antiquity: Studies in the Imagination of a Culture*. Princeton, NJ: Princeton University Press.

Miller, F. G., and Kaptchuk, T. J. (2008), 'The power of context: Reconceptualizing the placebo effect'. *Journal of the Royal Society of Medicine* 101 (5), 222–225.

https://doi.org/10.1258/jrsm.2008.070466.

Mills, H. (1984), 'Greek clothing regulations: Sacred and profane?' *Zeitschrift für Papyrologie und Epigraphik* 55, 255–265.

Mitchell, S. H., Laurent, C. L., and De Wit, H. (1996), 'Interaction of expectancy and the pharmacological effects of d-amphetamine: Subjective effects and self-administration'. *Psychopharmacology (Berl)* 125 (4), 371–378.

Mithen, S. (1996), *The Prehistory of the Mind: The Cognitive Origins of Art, Religion and Science*. London: Phoenix.

Mitropoulou, E. (1977), *Corpus I: Attic Votive Reliefs of the 6th and 5th Centuries B. C.* Athens: Pyli Editions.

Moerman, D. E. (1983), 'Perspectives on the placebo phenomenon'. *Medical Anthropology Quarterly* 14, 3–19.

Moerman, D. E. (2000), 'Cultural variations in the placebo effect: Ulcers, anxiety, and blood pressure'. *Medical Anthropology Quarterly* 14 (1), 51–72.

Moerman, D. E. (2002), *Meaning, Medicine and the Placebo Effect*. Cambridge: Cambridge University Press.

Molen, J. M. van der (2019), 'The language of Asclepius. The role and diffusion of the written word in – and the visual language of – the cult of Asclepius'. Retrieved from https://philarchive.org/rec/VANTLO-42.

Monroe, W. F., Holleman, W. L., and Holleman, M. C. (1992), 'Is there a person in this case?' *Literature and Medicine* 11 (1), 45–63.

Montgomery, G. H., and Kirsch, I. (1997), 'Classical conditioning and the placebo effect'. *Pain* 72, 107–113.

Morehouse, L. R. (2012), 'Dismemberment and devotion: Anatomical votive dedication in Italian popular religion'. *Honors Projects* 17. Retrieved from https://digitalcommons.macalester.edu/classics_honors/17

Morgan, M. H. (trans.) (1914), *Vitruvius. The Ten Books on Architecture*. Cambridge, MA: Harvard University Press.

Morris, C. (2009), 'Configuring the individual: Bodies of figurines in Minoan Crete'. In A. L. D'Agata and A. Van de Moortel (eds), *Archaeologies of Cult: Essays on Ritual and Cult in Crete in honor of Geraldine C. Gesell*. Hesperia (Suppl. 42). Princeton, NJ: American School of Classical Studies at Athens, pp. 179–187.

Morris, C., and Peatfield, A. A. D. (2014), 'Health and healing on Cretan Bronze Age peak sanctuaries'. In D. Michaelides (ed.), *Medicine and Healing in the Ancient Mediterranean World*. Oxford: Oxford University Press, pp. 54–63.

Morris, P. A. (1982), 'The effect of pilgrimage on anxiety, depression and religious attitude'. *Psychological Medicine* 12 (2), 291–294.

Muehlenbein, M. P., Hirschtick, J. L., Bonner, J. Z., and Swartz, A. M. (2010), 'Toward quantifying the usage costs of human immunity: Altered metabolic rates and hormone levels during acute immune activation in men'. *American Journal of Human Biology* 22 (4), 546–556.

Murphy, T. (2000), 'Discourse'. In W. Braun and R. McCutcheon (eds), *Guide to the*

Study of Religion. London: Bloomsbury, pp. 396–408.

Murray, A. T. (trans.) (1919), *The Odyssey*. London: W. Heinemann.

Musial, D. (1990), 'Sur le Culte d'Esculape à Rome et in Italie'. *Dyes in History and Archaeology* 16, 231–238.

Nakamura, R., and Fujii, E. (1992), 'A comparative study of the characteristics of the electroencephalogram when observing a hedge and a concrete block fence'. *Journal of the Japanese Institute of Landscape Architects* 55, 139–144.

Nayernouri, T. (2010), 'Asclepius, caduceus, and simurgh as medical symbols'. *Archives of Iranian Medicine* 13 (1), 61–68.

Neely, J. (1990), 'Semantic priming effects in visual word recognition: A selective review of current findings and theories'. In D. Besner and G. Humphreys (eds), *Basic Processing in Reading: Visual Word Recognition*. Hillsdale, NJ: Routledge, pp. 264–336.

Nesse, R. M. (1991), 'What good is feeling bad? The evolutionary utility of psychic pain'. *The Sciences* (November/December), pp. 30–37.

Nesse, R. M., and Williams, G. C. (1994), *Why We Get Sick: The New Science of Darwinian Medicine*. New York: Times Books.

Nesse, R. M., and Williams, G. C. (1998), 'Evolution and the origins of disease'. *Scientific American* 279, 86–93.

Nichols, D. E., and Chemel, R. B. (2006), 'The neuropharmacology of religious experience: Hallucinogens and the experience of the divine'. In P. McNamara (ed.), *Where God and Science Meet: How Brain and Evolutionary Studies Alter Our Understanding of Religion*. vol. 3. (Psychology, Religion and Spirituality). London: Praeger Perspectives, pp. 1–34.

Niklson, I., Edrich, P., and Verdru, P. (2006), 'Identifying baseline characteristics of placebo responders versus nonresponders in randomized double-blind trials of refractory partial-onset seizures'. *Epileptic Disorders* 8 (1), 37–44.

Nock, A. D. (1933), *Conversion: The Old and the New in Religion from Alexander the Great to Augustine of Hippo*. London: Oxford University Press.

Nordin, A. (2011), 'Dreaming in religion and pilgrimage: Cognitive, evolutionary and cultural perspectives'. *Religion* 41 (2), 225–249. https://doi.org/10.1080/0048721X.2011.553141.

Norman, D. A. (1993), *Things that Make Us Smart: Defending Human Attributes In The Age Of The Machine*. Reading, MA: Addison-Wesley.

Nowicki, K. (1994), 'Some remark on the pre- and protoplatial peak sanctuaries in Crete'. *Aegean Archaeology* 1, 31–48.

Nutton, V. (1977), 'Archiatri and the medical profession in antiquity'. *Papers of the British School at Rome* 45, 191–226. https://doi.org/10.1017/S0068246200009211.

Nutton, V. (1992), 'Healers in the medical market place: Towards a social history of Graeco-Roman medicine'. In A. Wear A. (ed.), *Medicine in Society: Historical Essays*. Cambridge: Cambridge University Press, pp. 15–58.

Nutton, V. (2005), *Ancient Medicine*. New York: Routledge.

Oberhelman, S. M. (1987), 'The diagnostic dream in ancient medical theory and practice'. *Bulletin of the history of medicine* 61 (1), 47-60.

Oberhelman, S. M. (2013), 'Introduction: Medical pluralism, healing, and dreams in Greek culture'. In S. M. Oberhelman (ed.), *Dreams, Healing, and Medicine in Greece: From Antiquity to the Present*. Farnham: Ashgate, pp. 1-32.

Oberhelman, S. M. (2014), 'Anatomical votive reliefs as evidence for specialization at healing sanctuaries in the ancient Mediterranean world'. *Athens Journal of Health* 1 (1), 47-62.

Ofshe, R. J. (1992), 'Inadvertent hypnosis during interrogation: False confession due to dissociative state: Mis-identified multiple personality and the satanic cult hypothesis'. *International Journal of Clinical and Experimental Hypnosis* 40 (3), 125-156. https://doi.org/10.1080/00207149208409653.

Oken, B. S. (2008), 'Placebo effects: Clinical aspects and neurobiology'. *Brain* 131 (pt.11), 2812-2823. https://doi.org/10.1093/brain/awn116.

O'Neill, E, Jr. (trans.) (1938), *Aristophanes. Wealth. The Complete Greek Drama, vol. 2*. New York: Random House.

Ong, L. M., De Haes, J. C., Hoos, A. M., and Lammes, F. B. (1995), 'Doctor-patient communication: A review of the literature'. *Social Science and Medicine* 40 (7), 903-918.

Orlin, E. M. (1997), *Temples, Religion and Politics in the Roman Republic*. Leiden: Brill.

Osborne, R. (2011) *The History Written on the Classical Body*. Cambridge: Cambridge University Press.

Ottosson, J., and Grahn, P. (2005), 'A comparison of leisure time spent in a garden with leisure time spent indoors: On measures of restoration in residents in geriatric care'. *Landscape Research* 30, 23-55. https://doi.org/10.1080/0142639042000324758.

Ousman, S. S., and P. Kubes (2012), 'Immune surveillance in the central nervous system'. *Nature Neuroscience* 15, 1096-1101. https://doi.org/10.1038/nn.3161.

Owens, I. P. F., and K. Wilson (1999), 'Immunocompetence: A neglected life history trait or a conspicuous red herring?'. *Trends in Evolution and Ecology* 14, 170-172. https://doi.org/10.1016/S0169-5347(98)01580-8

Pacheco-Lopez, G., Engler, H., Niemi, M. B., and Schedlowski, M. (2006), 'Expectations and associations that heal: Immunomodulatory placebo effects and its neurobiology'. *Brain, Behavior, and Immunity* 20, 430-446. https://doi.org/10.1016/j.bbi.2006.05.003.

Pacheco-Lopez, G., Niemi, M. B., Kou, W., Harting, M. et al. (2005), 'Neural substrates for behaviorally conditioned immunosuppression in the rat'. *Journal of Neuroscience* 25, 2330-2337. https://doi.org/10.1523/JNEUROSCI.4230-04.2005.

Pachis, P. (2003), *Isis Karpotokos, Oicoumene, Foreword to the syncretism of the Hellenistic*

age (in Greek), v. 1. Thessaloniki: Vanias.
Pachis, P. (2004), 'Foreword to the study of religions of the Hellenistic era' (in Greek). In H. L. Martin, *Religions of the Hellesnistic Era*. Translated by D. Xygalatas. Thessaloniki: Vanias, pp. 11–73.
Pachis, P. (2014), 'Dream and healing in the Isis/Sarapis cult during the Graeco-Roman Age'. *Journal of Cognitive Historiography* 1 (1), 52–71.
Pachis, P. and Panagiotidou, O. (2017), 'The long way from Cognitive Science to History: To shorten the distance and fill in the blanks'. In L. H. Martin and D. Wiebe (eds), *Religion Explained? The Cognitive Science of Religion after Twenty-Five Years*. London: Bloomsbury, pp. 89–96. https://doi.org/10.5040/9781350032491
Paton, W. R. (trans.) (1916), *The Greek Anthology*. London: W. Heinemann.
Panagiotidou, O. (2011), 'Divine healings at the temples of Asklepios as 'turning points' in the life narratives of supplicants'. *Proceedings of the 2nd Hellenistic Studies Workshop*. Alexandria: The Alexandria Center of Hellenistic Studies, pp. 124–136.
Panagiotidou, O. (2013), 'Location of an Asklepios' sanctuary: Why there? Why like that?'. Paper presented at Spatialising Practices: Landscapes, Mindscapes, Socioscapes: Towards a Redescriptive Companion to Graeco-Roman Antiquity, Loutraki, Greece, 23–27 June.
Panagiotidou, O. (2014a), 'Disease and healing in the Asclepius cult: A cognitive approach'. PhD dissertation, Aristotle University of Thessaloniki, Thessaloniki, Greece.
Panagiotidou, O. (2014b), 'The Asklepios cult: Where brains, minds and bodies interact with the world creating new realities'. *Journal of Cognitive Historiography* 1 (1), 14–23.
Panagiotidou, O. (2015), 'History meets cognition: The Asclepius cult as a pattern of practice'. Paper presented at XXI IAHR World Congress, Erfurt, Germany, 23-29 August.
Panagiotidou, O. (2016a), 'Religious healing and the Asclepius cult: A case of placebo effects'. *Open Theology* 2 (1), 79–91. https://doi.org/10.1515/opth-2016-0006
Panagiotidou, O. (2016b), 'Asclepius' myths and healing narratives: Counter-intuitive concepts and cultural expectations'. *Open Library of Humanities* 2 (1), e6, 1–26. https://doi.org/10.16995/olh.34
Panagiotidou, O. (2016c), 'Asclepius: A divine doctor, a popular healer'. In W. V. Harris (ed.), *Popular Medicine in Graeco-Roman Antiquity: Explorations*. (Columbia Studies in the Classical Tradition 42). Leiden: Brill.
Panagiotidou, O. (2018), 'Divination in Greek antiquity: Tracing divine signs in a world of expected and unexpected uncertainty'. *Pantheon* 13 (2), 3–26.
Panagiotidou, O. (2019), 'A biocultural approach to Aelius Aristides' *Sacred Tales*'. In A. Klostergaard Petersen, G. I. Sælid, L. H. Martin, J. S. Jensen

and J. Sørensen (eds), *Evolution, Cognition, and the History of Religion: A New Synthesis. Festschrift in Honour of Armin W. Geertz.* Leiden: Brill, pp. 506-523. https://doi.org/10.1163/9789004385375

Panagiotidou, O. (2021a), 'Emotional arousal, sensory deprivation and "miraculous healing" in the cult of Asclepius'. In D. Stein, S. K. Costello and K. Polinger Foster (eds), *Ecstatic Experience in the Ancient World.* Abingdon: Routledge, pp. 297-314.

Panagiotidou, O. (2021b), 'The placebo drama of the Asclepius Cult'. *Trends in Classics* 13 (1), 195-226.

Papachatzis, N. (2002), *Pausaniou Ellados Periegesis* (in Greek). Ekdotike Athenon: Athens.

Papaefthymiou, V. (2009), 'Der Altar des Asklepieions von Athen'. In J. T. Jensen, G. Hinge, P. Schultz and B. Wickkiser (eds,), *Aspects of Ancient Greek Cult Context, Ritual and Iconography.* (Aarhus Studies in Mediterranean Antiquity VIII). Aarhus: Aarhus University Press, pp. 67-89.

Parker, R. (1983), *Miasma. Pollution and Purification in Early Greek Religion*, Oxford: Clarendon Press.

Parker, R. (1985), 'Greek states and Greek oracles'. In P. A. Cartledge and F. D. Harvey (eds), *Crux: Essays in Greek History Presented to G. E. M. de Ste. Croix on his 75th Birthday, History of Political Thought 6½.* London: Duckworth Pub, pp. 76-108.

Parsons, T. (1951), *The Social System.* London: Routledge and Kegan Paul.

Parsons, T. (1958), 'Definitions of health and illness in the light of American values and social structure'. In E. G. Jaco (ed.), *Patients, Physicians and Illness: Sourcebook in Behavioral Science and Medicine.* New York: Free Press, pp. 165-187.

Parsons, T. (1964), *Social Structure and Personality.* New York: Free Press.

Patton, C. K. (2004), 'A great and strange correction: Intentionality, locality, and epiphany in the category of dream incubation'. *History of Religions* 43 (3), 194-223.

Pearcy, L. T. (2013), 'Writing the medical dream in the Hippocratic Corpus and at Epidaurus'. In S. M. Oberhelman (ed.), *Dreams, Healing, and Medicine in Greece: From Antiquity to the Present.* Farnham: Ashgate, pp.93-108.

Peatfield, A. A. D. (1990), 'Minoan peak sanctuaries: History and society'. *Opuscula Atheniensia* 18, 117-131.

Petrakos, C. V. (1968), *Oropos and the Sanctuary of Amphiaraos* (in Greek). Athens: Archaeological Society of Athens.

Petrakos, C. V. (1997), *The Inscriptions of Oropos* (in Greek). Athens: Archaeological Society of Athens.

Petridou, G. (2014), 'Asclepius the divine healer, Asclepius the divine physician: Epiphanies as diagnostic and therapeutic tools'. In D. Michaelides (ed.), *Medicine and Healing in the Ancient Mediterranean World.* Oxford: Oxbow

Books, pp. 291–301.

Petridou, G. (2016), *Divine Epiphany in Greek Literature and Culture*. Oxford: Oxford University Press.

Petridou, G. (2018), 'The curious case of Aelius Aristides. The author as sufferer and illness as "individualizing motif"'. In E.-M. Becker and J. Rüpke (eds), *Autoren in religiösen literarischen Texten der späthellenistischen und der frühkaiserzeitlichen Welt*. Tübingen: Mohr Siebeck, pp. 199–220.

Petrovic, A., and Petrovic, I. (2016), *Inner Purity and Pollution in Greek Religion: Volume I: Early Greek Religion*. Oxford: Oxford University Press.

Petrovic, P., Kalso, E., Peterson, K. M., and Ingvar, M. (2002), 'Placebo and opiod analgesia. Imaging a shared neuronal network'. *Science* 295, 1737–1740.

Petsalis-Diomidis, A. (2005), 'The body in space: Visual dynamics in Graeco-Roman healing pilgrimage'. In J. Elsner and I. Rutherford (eds), *Pilgrimage in Graeco-Roman and Early Christian Antiquity. Seeing the Gods*. Oxford: Oxford University Press, pp. 183–218.

Petsalis-Diomidis, A. (2006), 'Sacred writing, sacred reading: The function of Aelius Aristides' self-presentation as author in the *Sacred Tales*'. In J. Mossman and B. McGing (eds), *The Limits of Ancient Biography*. Swansea: Classical Press of Wales, pp. 193–211.

Petsalis-Diomidis, A. (2010), *Truly Beyond Wonders: Aelius Aristides and the Cult of Asklepios*. Oxford: Oxford University Press.

Phillips, E. D. (1952), 'A hypochondriac and his god'. *Greece and Rome* 21 (61), 23–36.

Pichot, P., Barucand, D., and Perse, J. (1967), 'L'attitude de l'aquiescement comme detirminant de l'effet placebo'. In J. Lassner (ed.), *Hypnosis and Psychosomatic Medicine. Proceedings of the International Congress for Hypnosis and Psychosomatic Medicine*, World Federation for Mental Health. Paris, April 1965. Amsterdam: Springer Verlag.

Piercy, M. A., Sramek, J. J., Kurtz, N. M., and Cutler, N. R. (1996), 'Placebo response in anxiety disorders'. *Annals of Pharmacotherapy* 30 (9), 1013–1019.

Pleket, H. W. (1983), 'Arts en maatshappij in het oude Griekenland: De sociale status van de arts'. *Tijdschrift voor Geschoedenis* 96, 325–347.

Pollo, A., Carlino, E., and Benedetti, F. (2008), 'The top-down influence of ergogenic placebos on muscle work and fatigue'. *European Journal of Neuroscience* 28, 379–388.

Pollo, A., Torre, E., Lopiano, L., Rizzone, M. et al. (2002), 'Expectation modulates the response to subthalamic nucleus stimulation in Parkinsonian patients'. *NeuroReport* 13, 1383–1386.

Porro, C. A. (2009), 'Open your mind to placebo conditioning'. *Pain* 145, 2–3.

Porubanova-Norquist, M., Shaw, D. J., and Xygalatas, D. (2013), 'Minimal counter-intuitiveness revisited: Effects of cultural and ontological violations on concept memorability'. *Journal for the Cognitive Science of Religion* 1 (2), 181–192. https://doi.org/10.1558/jcsr.v1i2.181

Porubanova-Norquist, M, Shaw, D J, McKay, R and Xygalatas, D. (2014), 'Memory for expectation-violating concepts: The effects of agents and cultural familiarity'. *PLoS ONE* 9(4): e90684. https://doi.org/10.1371/journal.pone.0090684

Potter, P. (ed. and trans.) (1995), *Hippocrates. Volume VIII*. Cambridge, MA: Harvard University Press.

Prêtre, C., and Charlier, P. (2009), *Maladies humaines, thérapies divines: Analyse épigraphique et paléopathologique de textes de guérison grecs*. (Archaiologia). M. Villeneuve-d'Ascq: Presses universitaires du Septentrion.

Price D. D., Milling L. S., Kirsch I., Duff A., Montgomery, G. H., and Nicholls, S. S. (1999), 'An analysis of factors that contribute to the magnitude of placebo analgesia in an experimental paradigm'. *Pain* 83 (2), 147–156.

Price, D. D., Finniss, D. G., and Benedetti, F. (2008), 'A comprehensive review of the placebo effect: Recent advances and current thought'. *Annual Review of Psychology* 59 (2), 1–226.

Prioreschi, P. (1992), 'Did the Hippocratic physician treat hopeless cases?' *Gesnerus* 49, 341–350.

Pulvermüller, F. (1999), 'Words in the brain's language'. *Behavioral and Brain Sciences* 22 (2), 253–336.

Purday, K. M. (1987), 'Minor healing cults within Athens and its environs'. PhD dissertation, University of Southampton, Southampton.

Purzycki, B. G., and Willard, A. K. (2016), 'MCI theory: A critical discussion'. *Religion, Brain and Behavior* 6 (3), 207–248.

Quincy, J. (1811), *Quincy's Lexicum-Medicum. A New Medical Dictionary*. Revised by R. Hooper. London.

Raafat, M. R., Chater, N., and Frith, C. (2009), 'Herding in humans'. *Trends in Cognitive Sciences* 13 (10), 420–428. https://doi.org/10.1016/j.tics.2009.08.002.

Rabkin, J. G., McGrath, P. J., Quitkin, F. M., Tricamo, E. et al. (1990), 'Effects of pill-giving on maintenance of placebo response in patients with chronic mild depression'. *American Journal of Psychiatry* 147, 1622–1626.

Randolph-Seng, B., and Nielsen, M. E. (2007), 'Honesty: One effect of primed religious representations'. *International Journal for the Psychology of Religion* 17 (4), 303–315. https://doi.org/10.1080/10508610701572812.

Randolph-Seng, B., and Nielsen, M. E. (2009), 'Opening the doors of perception: Priming altered states of consciousness outside of conscious awareness'. *Archive for the Psychology of Religion* 31 (2), 237–260. https://doi.org/10.1163/157361209X424475.

Renberg, G. H. (2006), 'Was incubation practiced in the Latin West?'. *Archiv für Religionsgeschichte* 8 (1), 105–148. https://doi.org/10.1515/9783110233834.105.

Renberg, G. H. (2006/2007), 'Public and private places of worship in the cult of Asclepius at Rome'. *Memoirs of the American Academy in Rome* 51/52, 87–172.

Renberg, G. H. (2010), 'Dream-narratives and unnarrated dreams in Greek and Latin dedicatory inscriptions'. In E. Scioli and C. Walde (eds), *Sub imagine somni: Nighttime Phenomena in the Greco-Roman World*. (Testi e studi di cultura classica 46). Pisa: Edizioni ETS, pp. 33–61.

Renberg, G. H. (2015), 'The role of dream-interpreters in Greek and Roman religion'. In G. Weber (ed.), *Artemidor von Daldis und die antike Traumdeutung: Texte - Kontexte - Lektüren*. (Colloquia Augustana 33). Berlin: W. De Gruyter, pp. 233–262.

Renberg, G. H. (2017), *Where Dreams May Come. Incubation Sanctuaries in the Greco-Roman World*. 2 vols. Leiden: Brill.

Renfrew, C., and Scarre, C. (eds) (1998), *Cognition and Material Culture: The Archaeology of Symbolic Storage*. Cambridge: McDonald Institute for Archaeological Research.

Rescorla, R. A. (1988), 'Pavlovian conditioning: It is not what you think it is'. *American Psychologist* 43 (3), 151–160. https://doi.org/10.1037//0003-066X.43.3.151.

Revonsuo, A. (1998), 'How to take consciousness seriously in cognitive neuroscience'. *Communication and Cognition* 30 (3–4), 185–205.

Riethmüller W. J. (2005), *Asklepios: Heiligtümer und Kulte*. 2 vols. (Studien zu Antiken Heiligtümern). Heidelberg: Verlag Archäologie und Geschichte.

Riley, H. T. (trans.) (1912), *The Comedies of Plautus*. London: G. Bell and Sons.

Rillo, A. (2008), 'The Greek origin of caduceum: Æsculapius'. *Colombia Médica* 39 (4), 384–388.

Rips, L. J. (1995), 'The current status of research on concept combination'. *Mind and Language* 10 (1–2), 72–104.

Robbins, P., and Aydede, M. (eds) (2009), *The Cambridge Handbook of Situated Cognition*. Cambridge: Cambridge University Press.

Roebuck, C. (1951), *The Asklepeion and Lerna, Cotinth. Results of Excavations conducted by the Americal School of Classical Studies at Athens*, vol. XIV. Princeton, NJ: The American School of Classical Studies at Athens.

Roepstorff, A., Niewöhner, J., and Beck, S. (2010), 'Enculturing brains through patterned practices'. *Neural Networks* 23 (8–9), 1051–1059. https://doi.org/10.1016/j.neunet.2010.08.002.

Roesch, P. (1982), 'Le Culte d'Asclepios à Rome'. In G. Sabbah (ed.), *Médecins et Médecine dans l'Antiquité*. (Centre Jean Palerne. Mémoires, III). Saint-Etienne: Publications de l'université de Saint-Etienne, pp. 171–179.

Rohde, E. (1925), *Psyche: The Cult of Souls and the Belief in Immortality among the Greeks*. Translated by H. B. Hillis. London: Routledge and Kegan Paul.

Roselli, A. (1996), *Ippocrate. La malattia sacra*. Venice: Marsilio.

Rossi, E. L., and Rossi, K. L. (2007), 'What is a suggestion? The neuroscience of implicit processing heuristics in therapeutic hypnosis and psychotherapy?'. *American Journal of Clinical Hypnosis* 49 (4), 267–281.

Rostovtzeff, M. I. (1941), *The Social and Economic History of the Hellenistic World*.

Oxford: Oxford University Press.

Roux, G. (1961), *L'architecture de l'Argolide aux IVe et IIIe siècles avant J.-C.* Paris: de Boccard.

Rowlands, M. (2003), *Externalism: Putting Mind and World Back Together Again.* Chesham: Acumen.

Rublack, U. (2013), 'Matter in the material renaissance'. *Past and Present* 219, 41–85.

Ruffle, B., and Sosis, R. (2010), 'Do religious contexts elicit more trust and altruism? An experiment on Facebook'. *Social Science Research Network* 1566123. https://doi.org/10.2139/ssrn.1566123.

Russell, D. A., Trapp, M., and H.-G. Nesselrath (eds) (2016), *In Praise of Asclepius. Aelius Aristides, Selected Prose Hymns.* Tübingen: Mohr Siebeck.

Rynearson, N. (2003), 'Constructing and deconstructing the body in the cult of Asklepios'. *Stanford Journal of Archaeology.* Retrieved from www.stanford.edu/dept/archaeology/journal/newdraft/2003_Journal/rynearson/paper.pdf (accessed 31 January 2012).

Sachs, L. (1988), *Medicinsk Antropologi.* Stockholm: Liber.

Sahlas, D. (2001), 'Functional neuroanatomy in the pre-Hippocratic era: Observations from the Iliad of Homer'. *Neurosurgery* 48 (6), 1352-1357.

Salazar, C. F. (2000), *The Treatment of War Wounds in Greco-Roman Antiquity.* Leiden: Brill.

Samama, É. (2003), *Les médecins dans le monde grec: Sources épigraphiques sur la naissance d'un corps médical.* Geneva: Librairie Droz.

Santos, G. H. (2000), 'Chest trauma during the battle of Troy: Ancient warfare and chest trauma'. *The Annals of Thoracic Surgery* 69 (4), 1285-1287.

Scarborough, J. (1991), 'Pharmacology of sacred plants, herbs, and roots'. In C. A. Faraone and D. Obbink (eds), *Magika Hiera: Ancient Greek Magic and Religion.* Oxford: Oxford University Press, pp. 138-174.

Schachter, A. (1981), *Cults of Boiotia.* 4 vols. London: University of Oxford.

Schacter, L. D., Dobbins, G. I., and Schnyer, M. D. (2004), 'Specificity of priming: A cognitive neuroscience perspective'. *Nature Reviews, Neuroscience* 5, 853–862. https://doi.org/10.1038/nrn1534.

Schäfer, D. (2000), 'Traum und Wunderheilung im Asklepios-Kult in der griechisch-römische Medizin'. In A. Karenberg and C. Leitz (eds), *Heilkunde und Hochkultur, I: Geburt, Seuche, und Traumdeutung in den antiken Zivilisation des Mittelmeerraumes.* (Naturwissenschaft – Philosophie – Geschichte 14). Hamburg: LIT, pp. 268-272.

Schlange-Schöningen, H. (2001), *Die römische Gesellschaft bei Galen. Biographie und Sozialgeschichte.* Habilitationschrift: Freie Universität Berlin.

Schofield, M. (1986), 'Cicero for and against divination'. *Journal of Roman Studies* 76, 47–65.

Schörner, G. (2015), 'Anatomical ex votos'. In R. Raja and J. Rüpke (eds), *A Companion to the Archaeology of Religion in the Ancient World.* (Blackwell Companions to

the Ancient World). Chichester: Wiley-Blackwell, pp. 397-411.
Schultz, W. (2006), 'Behavioral theories and the neurophysiology of reward'. *Annual Review of Psychology* 57, 87-115.
Schultz, W. (2008), 'Introduction. Neuroeconomics: The promise and the profit'. *Philosophical Transactions of the Royal Society B: Biological Sciences* 363 (1511), 3767-3769.
Schweinhardt, P., Seminowicz, D. A., Jaeger, E., Duncan, G. H. et al. (2009), 'The anatomy of the mesolimbic reward system: A link between personality and the placebo analgesic response'. *Journal of Neuroscience* 29, 4882-4887.
Schweizer, E., and Rickels, K. (1997). 'Placebo response in generalized anxiety: Its effect on the outcome of clinical trials'. *Journal of Clinical Psychiatry* 58 (Suppl. 11), 30-38.
Scott, D. J., Stohler, C. S., Egnatuk, C. M., Wang, H. et al. (2007), 'Individual differences in reward responding explain placebo-induced expectations and effects'. *Neuron* 55, 325-336.
Scott, D. J., Stohler, C. S., Egnatuk, C. M., Wang, H. et al. (2008), 'Placebo and nocebo effects are defined by opposite opioid and dopaminergic responses'. *Archives of General Psychiatry* 65, 1225-1226.
Seibert, J. (1979), *Die politischen Flüchtlinge und Verbannten in der griechischen Geschichter von den Anfängen bis zur Unterwerfung durch die Römer*. 2 vols. Sarmstadt: Wissenschaftliche Buchgesellschaft.
Semeria, A. (1986), 'Per un censimento degli Asklepieia della Grecia continentale e delle Isole'. *Annali della Scuola Normale Superiore di Pisa. Classe di Lettere e Filosofia Serie III* 16 (4), 931-958.
Shanks, D. R. (2010), 'Learning: From association to cognition'. *Annual Review of Psychology* 61, 273-301.
Shapiro, A. K. (1963), 'Psychological aspects of medication'. In H. I. Lief, V. F. Lief and N. R. Lief (eds), *The Psychological Basis of Medical Practice*. New York: Hoeber.
Shapiro, A. K. (1964), 'A historic and heuristic definition of the placebo'. *Psychiatry* 27, 52-58.
Shapiro, A. K. (1969), 'Iatroplacebogenics'. *International Pharmacopsychiatry* 2, 215-248.
Shapiro, A. K., and Shapiro, E. (1997a), *The Powerful Placebo: From Ancient Priest to Modern Physician*. Baltimore, MD: Johns Hopkins University Press.
Shapiro, A. K., and Shapiro, E. (1997b), 'The placebo: Is it much ado about nothing?'. In A. Harrington (ed.), *The Placebo Effect: An Interdisciplinary Exploration*. Cambridge, MA: Harvard University Press, pp. 12-36.
Shariff, A., and Norenzayan, A. (2007), 'God is watching you: Priming god concepts increases prosocial behavior in an anonymous economic game'. *Psychological Science* 18 (9), 803-809. https://doi.org/10.1111/j.1467-9280.2007.01983.x.

Sheldon, B. C., and Verhulst, S. (1996), 'Ecological immunology: Costly parasite defences and tradeoffs in evolutionary ecology'. *Trends in Ecology and Evolution* 11, 317–321.

Sherwin-White, S. M. (1978), *Ancient Cos*. Göttingen: Vandenhoeck und Ruprecht.

Shipley, G., and Hansen, M. (2006), 'The polis and federalism'. In Bugh G. R. (ed.), *The Cambridge Companion to the Hellenistic World*. (Cambridge Companions to the Ancient World). Cambridge: Cambridge University Press, pp. 52–72.

Siefert, H. (1980), 'Inkubation, Imagination und Kommunikation im antiken Asklepioskult'. In Leuner, H. (ed.), *Katathymes Bilderleben. Ergebnisse in Theorie und Praxis*. Bern: Huber, pp. 324–345.

Siegel, S. (2002), 'Explanatory mechanisms for placebo effects: Pavlovian conditioning'. In H. A. Guess, A. Kleinman, J. W. Kusek and L. W. Engel (eds), *The science of the placebo*. London: BMJ Books, pp. 133–157.

Simmons, K., and Barsalou, L. W. (2003), 'The similarity-in-topography principle: Reconciling theories of conceptual deficits'. *Cognitive Neuropsychology* 20, 451–486.

Singer, P. N. (1997), *Galen. Selected Works*. Oxford: Oxford University Press.

Sisti, D., and Caplan, A. (2017), 'The concept of disease'. In M. Solomon, J. E. Simon, and H. Kincaid (2017), *The Routledge Companion to Philosophy of Medicine*. (Routledge Philosophy Companions). New York: Routledge, pp. 5–15.

Slingerland, E. (2014), 'Toward a second wave of consilience in the cognitive scientific study of religion'. *Journal of Cognitive Historiography* 1 (1), 121–130.

Smith, R. C. (1986), 'Evaluating dream function: Emphasizing the study of patients with organic disease'. *The Journal of Mind and Behavior* 7, 397–410.

Smith, W. D. (1990), *Hippocrates. Pseudepigraphic Writings. Letters-Embassy-Speech from the Altar-Decree*. (Studies in Ancient Medicine, 2). Leiden: Brill.

Snyder, C. R. (1994), *The Psychology of Hope: You Can Get There from Here*. New York: Free Press.

Snyder, C. R., Harris, C., Anderson, J. R., Holleran, S. A., Irving, L. M., Sigmon, S. T., Yoshinobu, L., Gibb, J., Langelle, C., and Harney, P. (1991), 'The will and the ways: Development and validation of an individual-differences measure of hope'. *Journal of Personality and Social Psychology* 60 (4), 570–585.

Snyder, C. R., Hardi, S. S., Cheavens, J., Michael, S. T., Yamhure, L., and Sympson, S. (2000), 'The role of hope in cognitive behavior therapies'. *Cognitive Therapy and Research* 24 (6), 747–776. https://doi.org/10.1023/A:1005547730153

Sokolowski, F. (1973), 'On the new Pergamene lex sacra'. *Greek, Roman, and Byzantine Studies* 14 (4), 407–413.

Solomon, M., Simon, J. E., and Kincaid, H. (2017), *The Routledge Companion to Philosophy of Medicine*. (Routledge Philosophy Companions). New York: Routledge.

Spanos, N. P., Burgess, C. A., Burgess, M. F., Samuels, C., and Blois, W. O. (1998), 'Creating false memories of infancy with hypnotic and non-hypnotic procedures'. *Applied Cognitive Psychology* 13 (3), 201–218. https://doi.org/10.1002/(SICI)1099-0720(199906)13:3<201::AID-ACP565>3.0.CO;2-X

Sperber, D. (1996), *Explaining Culture: A Naturalistic Approach*. London: Blackwell.

Stafford, E. (2005), '"Without you no one is happy": The cult of Health in ancient Greece'. In H. King (ed.), *Health in Antiquity*. London, New York: Routledge, pp. 120–135.

Stannard, J. (1982), 'Medicinal plants and folk remedies in Pliny, "Historia Naturalis"'. *History and Philosophy of the Life Sciences* 4 (1), 3–23.

Steger, F. (2018), *Asclepius. Medicine and Cult*. Translated by M. M. Saar. Stuttgart: Franz Steiner Verlag.

Stephens, J. C. (2012), 'The dreams of Aelius Aristides: A psychological interpretation', *International Journal of Dream Research* 5 (1), 76–86.

Sternbach, R. A. (1964), 'The effects of instructional sets on autonomic responsivity'. *Psychophysiology* 62, 67–72.

Stewart, M. A. (1995), 'Effective physician–patient communication and health outcomes: A review'. *Canadian Medical Association Journal* 152, 423–433.

Stich, S. (1983), *From Folk Psychology to Cognitive Science*. (New Problems of Philosophy 9). Cambridge, MA: MIT Press.

Stockhorst, U., Gritzmann, E., Klopp, K., Schottenfeld-Naor, Y. Hübinger A, Berresheim, H. W., Steingrüber, H. J., and Gries, F. A. (1999), 'Classical conditioning of insulin effects in healthy humans'. *Psychosomatic Medicine* 61, 424–435.

Stockhorst, U., Steingruber, H. J., and Scherbaum, W. A. (2000), 'Classically conditioned responses following repeated insulin and glucose administration in humans'. *Behavioral Brain Research* 110, 143–159.

Stoneman, R. (2011), *The Ancient Oracles: Making the Gods Speak*. New Haven, CT: Yale University Press.

Storbeck, J., and Clore, G. L. (2008), 'The affective regulation of cognitive priming'. *Emotion* 8 (2), 208–215. https://doi.org/10.1037/1528-3542.8.2.208.

Strange, P. G. (1992), *Brain Biochemistry and Brain Disorders*. New York: Oxford University Press.

Strauss, C., and Quinn, N. (1997), *A Cognitive Theory of Cultural Meaning*. Cambridge, MA: Cambridge University Press.

Styrt, B., and Sugarman, B. (1990), 'Antipyresis and fever'. *Archives of Internal Medicine* 150, 1589–1597.

Susser, M. (1973), *Causal Thinking in the Health Sciences*. New York: Oxford University Press.

Sutton, J., and Keene, N. (2015), 'Cognitive history and material culture'. In D. Gaimster, T. Hamling and C. Richardson (eds), *The Ashgate Research Companion to Material Culture in Early Modern Europe*. (Ashgate Research Companions). Farnham: Ashgate, pp. 44–58.

Svenaeus, F. (2014), 'What is phenomenology of medicine? Embodiment, illness and being-in-the-world'. In H. Carel and R. Cooper (eds), *Health, Illness and Disease: Philosophical Essays*. London: Routledge.

Svensson, E., Råbrg, L., Koch, C., and Hasselquist, D. (1998), 'Energetic stress, immunosuppression and the costs of an antibody response'. *Functional Ecology* 12, 912–919.

Tagliabue, A. (2016), 'An embodied reading of epiphanies in Aelius Aristides' Sacred Tales'. *Ramus* 45 (2), 213–230. https://doi.org/10.1017/rmu.2016.11

Taylor, T. (ed. and trans.) (1821), *Iamblichus on the Mysteries of the Egyptians, Chaldeans, and Assyrians*. London: C. Whittingham.

Taylor, T. (ed. and trans.) (1823), *Select Works of Porphyry; Containing his Four Books on Abstinence from Animal Food; his Treatise On the Homeric Cave of the Nymphs; and his Auxiliaries to the Perception of Intelligible Natures*. London: T. Rodd.

Temkin, O. (1971), *The Falling Sickness. A History of Epilepsy from the Greeks to the Beginnings of Modern Neurology*. Baltimore, MD: Johns Hopkins University Press.

Temkin, O. (1973), *Galenism. Rise and Decline of a Medical Philosophy*. Ithaca, NY: Cornell University Press.

Temkin, O. (1991), *Hippocrates in a World of pagan and Christians*. Baltimore, MD: Johns Hopkins University.

Themelis, P. (2010), 'The asklepieion of Messene' (in Greek). *Deltos* 40, 5–25.

Tibbets, R. W., and Hawking, J. R. (1956), 'The placebo response'. *Journal of Medical Sciences* 102, 60–66.

Tick, E. (2001), *The Practice of Dream Healing: Bringing Ancient Greek Mysteries into Modern Medicine*. Wheaton: Quest Books.

Travlos, J. (1971), *Pictorial Dictionary of Ancient Athens*. London: Thames and Hudson.

Turk, D. C., and Genest, M. (1979), 'Regulation of pain: The application of cognitive and behavioural techniques for prevention and remediation'. In P. C. Kendall (ed.), *Cognitive-Behavioral Interventions: Theory, Research, and Procedures*. New York: Academic Press, pp. 287–319.

Turk, D. C., Meichenbaum, D., and Genest, M. (1987), *Pain and Behavioral Medicine: A Cognitive-Behavioral Perspective*. New York: Guilford Press.

Turkkan, J. S., and Brady, J. V. (1985), 'Mediational theory of the placebo effect'. In L. White, B. Tursky and G. E. Schwartz (eds), *Placebo: Theory, Research and Mechanisms*. New York: Guilford Press, pp. 324–331.

Turner, J. A., Deyo, R. A., Loeser, J. D., Von Korff, M., and Fordyce, W. E. (1994), 'The importance of placebo effects in pain treatment and research'. *Journal of the American Medical Association* 271 (20), 1609–1614.

Twaddle, A. (1968), 'Influence and illness: Definitions and definers of illness behavior among older males in Providence, Rhode Island'. PhD dissertation, Brown University, Providence, RI.

Twaddle, A. (1994), 'Disease, illness and sickness revisited'. In A. Twaddle and L. Nordenfelt (eds), *Disease, Illness and Sickness: Three Central Concepts in the*

Theory of Health. (Studies on Health and Society 18). Linköping: Linköping University, pp. 1–18.

Uhlenhuth, E. H., Rickels, K., Fisher, S., Park, L. C., Lipman, R. S., and Mock, J. (1966), 'Drug, doctor's verbal attitude and clinic setting in the symptomatic response to pharmacotherapy'. *Psychopharmacologia* 9, 392–418.

Ulrich, R. S. (1981), 'Natural versus urban scenes. Some psychological effects'. *Environment and Behavior* 13, 523–556.

Ulrich, R. S. (1984), 'View through a window may influence recovery from surgery'. *Science* 224 (4647), 420–421.

Ulrich, R. S. (1999), 'Effects of gardens on health outcomes: Theory and research'. In C. Cooper-Marcus and M. Barnes (eds), *Healing Gardens: Therapeutic Benefits and Design Recommendations*. New York: Wiley, pp. 27–86.

Ulrich, R. S. (2002), 'Health benefits of gardens in hospitals'. Retrieved from: http://plantsolutions.com/documents/HealthSettingsUlrich.pdf (accessed 2 August 2013).

Ulrich, R. S., Simons, R. F., Losito, B. D., Fiorito, E., Miles, M. A., and Zelson, M. (1991), 'Stress recovery during exposure to natural and urban environments'. *Journal of Environmental Psychology* 11 (3), 201–230.

Usener, H. (1896), *Götternamen. Versuch einer Lehre von der Religiösen Begriffsbildung*. Bonn: F. Cohen.

Ustinova, Y. (2009), 'Apollo Iatros: A Greek god of Pontic origin'. In K. Stähler and G. Gudrian (eds), *Griechen und ihre Nachbarn am Nordrand des Schwarzen Meers*. Münster: Ugarit-Verlag, pp. 245–299.

Ustinova, Y. (2013), 'Modes of prophecy, or modern arguments in support of the ancient approach'. *Kernos* 26, 25–44.

Van der Eijk, P. J. (2005), *Medicine and Philosophy in Classical Antiquity: Doctors and Philosophers on Nature, Soul, Health and Disease*. Cambridge: Cambridge University Press.

Van der Ploeg, G. E. (2018). *The Impact of the Roman Empire on the Cult of Asclepius*. (Impact of Empire XXX). Leiden: Brill.

Van Straten, F. T. (1981), 'Gifts for the gods'. In H. S. Versnel (ed.), *Faith, Hope and Worhsip*. Leiden: Brill, pp. 65–151.

Van Straten, F. T. (1992), 'Votives and votaries in Greek sanctuaries'. In A. Schachter, J. Bingen, and F. Hardt (eds), *Le sanctuaire grec: huit exposés suivis de discussions*. Geneva: Fondation Hardt, pp. 247–284.

Velarde, M. D., Fryb, G., and Tveitb, M. (2007), 'Health effects of viewing landscapes – Landscape types in environmental psychology'. *Urban Forestry and Urban Greening* 6, 199–212.

Verbanck-Piérard, A. (2000), 'Les héros guérisseurs: des dieux comme les autres'. In V. Pirenne-Delforge, and E. Suárez de la Torre (eds), *Héros et héroïnes dans les mythes et les cultes grecs. Actes du colloque de Valladolid*. Liège: Centre International d'Etude de la Religion Grecque Antique, pp. 281–332.

Vernant, J. P. (1991), 'Mortals and immortals: The body of the divine corps obscure'. In F. I. Zeitlin (ed.), *Mortals and Immortals: Collected Essays*. Princeton, NJ: Princeton University Press, pp. 27–49.
Versnel, H. S. (1981), 'Religious mentality in ancient prayer'. In H. S. Versnel (ed.), *Faith, Hope and Worhsip*. Leiden: Brill, pp. 1–64.
Versnel, H. S. (2011), *Coping with the Gods: Wayward Readings in Greek Theology*. Leiden: Brill. https://doi.org/10.1163/ej.9789004204904.i-594.
Veyne, P. (1988), *Did the Greeks Believe in Their Myths? An Essay on the Constitutive Imagination*. Translated by P. Wissing. Chicago, IL: University of Chicago Press.
Vikela, E. (2006), 'Healer gods and healing sanctuaries in Attica: Similarities and differences'. *Archiv für Religionsgeschichte* 8, 41–62.
Vits, S., and Schedlowski, M. (2014), 'Learned placebo effects in the immune system'. *Zeitschrift für Psychologie* 222 (3), 148–153.
Vits, S., Cesko, E., Enck, P., Hillen, U., Schadendorf, D., and Schedlowski, M. (2011), 'Behavioural conditioning as the mediator of placebo responses in the immune system'. *Philosophical Transactions of the Royal Society B: Biological Sciences* 366 (1572), 1799–1807.
Von Ehrenheim, H. (2015), *Greek Incubation Rituals in Classical and Hellenistic Times*. (Kernos Suppl. 29). Liège: Presses Universitaires de Liège.
Von Staden, H. (1990), 'Incurability and hopelessness: The Hippocratic corpus'. In P. Potter, G. Maloney, and J. Désautels (eds), *La maladie et les maladies dans la Collection hippocratique: Actes du VIe colloque international Hippocratique*. Québec: Éditions du Sphinx, pp. 75–112
Voudouris, N. J., Peck. C. L., and Coleman, G. (1985) 'Conditioned placebo responses'. *Journal of Personality and Social Psychology* 48 (1), 47–53.
Voudouris, N. J., Peck. C. L., and Coleman, G. (1990), 'The role of conditioning and verbal expectancy in the placebo response'. *Pain* 43 (1), 121–128.
Wager, T. D., Scott, D. J., and Zubieta, J. K. (2006), 'Placebo effects on human μ-opioid activity during pain'. *Proceedings of the National Academy of Sciences of the United States of America* 104 (26), 11056–11061. https://doi.org/10.1073/pnas.0702413104.
Wager, T. D., Billing, J. K., Smith, E. E., Sokolik, A., Casey, K. L., Davidson, R. J., Kosslyn, S. M., Rose, R. M., and Cohen, J. D. (2004), 'Placebo-induced changes in fMRI in the anticipation and experience of pain'. *Science* 303, 1162–1166.
Walbank, F. (1999), *The Hellenistic World* (in Greek). Translated by T. Darveris. Vanias: Thessaloniki.
Warrington, E. K., and McCarthy, R. A. (1987), 'Categories of knowledge: Further fractionations and an attempted integration'. *Brain* 110, 1273–1296.
Webster, T. B. L. (1954), 'Personification as a mode of Greek thought'. *Journal of the Warburg and Courtauld Institutes* 17 (1/2), 10–21.
Weil, A. (1995), *Spontaneous Healing How to Discover and Embrace Your Body's Natural*

Ability to Maintain and Heal Itself. London: Warner Books.
Welch, W. J. (1972), *What Happened in Between: A Country Doctor in Princeton.* New York: Braziller.
Wells, L. (1998) *The Greek Language of Healing from Homer to New Testament Times.* Berlin: W. De Gruyter.
White, L. M. (1990), *Building God's House in the Roman World: Architectural Adaptation Among Pagans, Jews, and Christians.* Baltimore, MD: Johns Hopkins University Press.
Whitehouse, H. (2004), *Modes of Religiosity: A Cognitive Theory of Religious Transmission.* Walnut Creek, CA: AltaMira Press.
Wickkiser, B. L. (2008), *Asklepios, Medicine, and the Politics of Healing in Fifth-Century Greece: Between Craft and Cult.* Baltimore, MD: Johns Hopkins University Press.
Wickkiser, B. L. (2009), 'Banishing plague: Asklepios, Athens, and the great plague reconsidered'. In J. T. Jensen, G. Hinge, P. Schultz and B. Wickkiser (eds), *Aspects of Ancient Greek Cult Context, Ritual and Iconography.* (Aarhus Studies in Mediterranean Antiquity VIII). Aarhus: Aarhus University Press, pp. 56–65.
Wickramasekera, I. (1980), 'A conditioned response model of the placebo effect predictions from the model'. *Biofeedback and Self-Regulation* 5 (1), 5–18.
Wiech, K., Farias, M., Kahane, G., Shackel, N. Tiede, W., and Tracey, I. (2008), 'An fMRI study measuring analgesia enhanced by religion as a belief system'. *Pain* 139 (2), 467–476.
Wilkins, W. (1985), 'Placebo controls and concepts in chemotherapy and psychotherapy research'. In L. White, B. Tursky and G. E. Schwartz (eds), *Placebo: Theory, Research and Mechanisms.* New York: Guilford Press, pp. 83–109.
Williams, A. (ed.) (1999), *Therapeutic Landscapes: The Dynamic between Place and Wellness.* New York: University Press of America.
Wilson, M. (2010), 'The re-tooled mind: How culture re-engineers cognition'. *Social, Cognitive, and Affective Neuroscience* 5 (2–3), 180–187.
Wisniewski, E. J. (1997), 'When concepts combine'. *Psychonomic Bulletin and Review* 4 (2), 167–183.
Wöhlers, M. (1999), *Heilige Krankheit. Epilepsie in antiker Medizin, Astrologie und Religion.* Marburg: N. G. Elwert.
Wolf, S., Doering, C. R., Clark, M. L., and Hagans, J. A. (1957), 'Chance distribution and the placebo "reactor"'. *Journal of Laboratory and Clinical Medicine* 49, 837–841.
Woods, S. C. (1972), 'Conditioned hypoglycemia: Effect of vagotomy and pharmacological blockade'. *American Journal of Physiology* 223, 1424–1427.
Woods, S. C., Makous, W., and Hutton, R. A. (1968), 'A new technique for conditioned hypoglycemia'. *Psychonomic Science* 10, 389–390.
Woods, S. C., Makous, W., and Hutton, R. A. (1969), 'Temporal parameters of

conditioned hypoglycemia'. *Journal of Comparative and Physiological Psychology* 69, 301–307.

Wroth, W. (1882), *Apollo with the Aesculapian Staff.* London: Taylor and Walton.

Xygalatas, D. (2006), 'An introduction to the cognitive study of religion' (in Greek). In H. Whitehouse, *Modes of Religiosity: A Cognitive Theory of Religious Transmission* (in Greek). Translated by D. Xygalatas. Thessaloniki: Vanias, pp. 9–87.

Xygalatas, D. (2012), *The Burning Saints: Cognition and Culture in the Fire-Walking Rituals of the Anastenaria.* London: Equinox.

Xygalatas, D., Schjoedt, U., Bulbulia, J., Konvalinka, I., Jegindø, E.-M., Reddish, P. et al. (2013). 'Autobiographical memory in a fire-walking ritual'. *Journal of Cognition and Culture* 13 (1), 1–16.

Xygalatas, D. (in press), 'Evil eyes and baking pies: Aspects of Greek divination, past and present'. In A. Klostergaard Petersen, and J. Sørensen (eds), *Divination and Magic and Their Interactions Empirical and Theoretical Perspectives.* (Numen Book Series). Leiden: Brill.

Zahn, R., Moll, J., Iyengar, V., Huey, E. D., Tierney, M., Krueger, F., and Grafman, J. (2009), 'Social conceptual impairments in frontotemporal lobar degeneration with right anterior temporal hypometabolism'. *Brain* 132 (3), 604–616. https://doi.org/10.1093/brain/awn343.

Zhang, W., Robertson, J., Jones, A. C., Dieppe, P. A. et al. (2008), 'The placebo effect and its determinants in osteoarthritis: Meta-analysis of randomised controlled trials'. *Annals of the Rheumatic Diseases* 67, 1716–1723.

Ziegenaus, O., and De Luca, G. (1968), *Das Asclepeio. Der südliche Temenosbezirk in hellenistischer und frührömischer Zeit.* Berlin: W. De Gruyter.

Ziehen, J. (1892), 'Über die Lage des Asklepiosheiligtums von Trikka'. *Athenische Mitteilungen* 17, 195–197.

Zollman, C., and Vickers, A. (1999), 'ABC of complementary medicine. Complementary medicine and the patient'. *British Medical Journal* 319, 1486–1489.

Zubieta, J. K., Bueller, J. A., Jackson, L. R., Scott, D. J. et al. (2005), 'Placebo effects mediated by endogenous opioid activity on m-opioid receptors'. *Journal of Neuroscience* 25, 7754–7762.

Zubieta, J. K., Yau, W. Y., Scott, D. J., and Stohler, C. S. (2006), 'Belief or need? Accounting for individual variations in the neurochemistry of the placebo effect'. *Brain, Behavior, and Immunity* 20, 15–26.

Zunino, M. L. (1997), *Hiera Messeniaka. La Storia religiosa della Messenia dall'Età micenea all'Età hellenistica.* Udine: Forum.

Index

Aceso 46, 103
acetylcholine, cholinergic neurochemical 137
Achelous 79
Acragas 74
adaptive error(s) 84, 85, 157
Admetus 41
Aegle 46
Aeschines 76, 85
Aesculapius 73, 77, 78, 97, 126
Africa 74, 102
agency 45, 62, 93, 94, 159
agents
    of dissemination 74
    historical 5, 160
    human 15, 153, 154, 159, 160
    human-like 43, 44, 61
    non-human 42, 62
    religious 43
    superhuman 7, 42, 43
    supernatural 7, 62
agentic thinking 92, 93
Aigina 69, 106, 125
Aleshire, B. S. 70
Alexander the Great 71
Alexandria 71
altered state(s) of consciousness 18, 63, 124, 143, 144, 145, 151, 158
Ambrosia from Athens 84, 85, 111
aminergic modulation (in the brain) 137
aminergic neurochemicals (serotonin and norepinepherine) 137
Amphiaraos 49
Amynos 49
Anaphe 73
anthropomorphism 42, 43, 61, 62
antibody production 28, 29
Antiocheia 71
Antiochos 71
anxiety 7, 15, 23, 30, 34, 82, 84, 93, 118, 129, 130
anxiety disorder(s) 28
Apollo 39–41, 42, 44, 46, 48, 63, 69, 71, 79, 98, 103, 141
    Apollo Iatros 48
    Apollo Kyparissios 80
    Apollo Maleatas 69, 77, 79
Apollophanes 70
Arcadia 69, 70, 72
Argos 69, 72
Aristophanes 86
Aristophanes' *Plutus* 125
Arnobius 97
Arsinoë 39, 40, 70
Artemidorus 65
Artemis 39, 40, 44, 48, 77
artisans 109
Asclepiades 50, 99
Asclepian therapy 18, 117, 134
asclepieion 3, 67, 68, 82, 92, 93, 102, 110, 122, 123

asclepieia, great 1, 17, 67, 75–77, 79, 81, 98, 101, 153
asclepieion in Athens/Athenian asclepieion/asclepieion on the Acropolis 50, 70, 52, 120
asclepieion in Cibyra 53
asclepieion of Aigina 125
asclepieion of Epidaurus/Epidaurian asclepieion/Epidaurian sanctuary 2, 46, 76, 77, 78, 79, 98, 106, 109, 113, 124
asclepieion of Kos/Koan asclepieion 51, 69, 71, 77, 80, 94, 95, 96
asclepieion of Lebena 70, 77, 79, 113
asclepieion of Pergamum/Pergamene asclepieion 70, 76, 77, 98, 114
asclepieion of Piraeus 50, 125, 132
asclepieion of Tiber Island/Roman asclepieion 73
asclepieion, Messenian 74
Asia Minor 1, 48, 52, 70, 71, 73, 127
Askitopoulou, Helen 126, 140
asthma 28
Athena 40, 44, 48
Athenians 70, 97
attention reinforcement 156
attention, regulation of 138
Attica 72
authority
    Asclepius'/god's 86, 89, 155, 156
    of doctors 27, 55
    external 35
    trust in 29

Balagrae in Cyrenaica 74, 102
baldness 114
balkanization 7
Bandura, Albert 100
Barsalou, Laurence 19, 146, 147
Berridge, Kent C. 17, 107
Berytus 73

biocultural approach 140
biocultural theory 11, 14
Bithynia 73
bizarreness (dreaming) 137, 141, 151
Black Sea 48
blind(ness) 84, 106, 110, 111
bloodletting 27
body fragmentation 119, 121, 122
Bosinelly, Marino 18, 139
Boyer, Pascal 7, 37, 42–43, 47, 62, 111, 157
brain activity 81, 137
brain regions 10, 88
    adjacent (parastriate) regions 137
    amygdala 31, 88
    anterior cingulate cortex 27, 138
    association areas 147–148
    cerebral cortex 27
    dorsal horn neurons 27
    dorsal striatum 31
    dorsolateral prefrontal cortex 27
    forebrain structures 107
    frontal cortex 88
    hippocampus 88
    hypothalamus 27
    insular cortex 31
    limbic system 137
    neostriatum 107
    nucleus accumbens 27, 107
    prefrontal cortex 27, 87, 137
    occipital lobe 137
    parastriate area 137
    periaqueductal gray 27
    primary visual cortex 137
    right parietal lobe 138
    rostroventromedial medulla 27
    spinal cord 27
    substantia nigra 31, 107
    subthalamic nucleus 31
    ventral striatum 87, 88
    ventral tegmental area/ventral tegmentum 27, 107

ventromedial hypothalamic
   nucleus 31
ventromedial prefrontal cortex 87
brain structures 9, 10
brain-immunity effects 29
Bronze Age 48, 49,
Bulbulia, Joseph 84

caduceus 44, 45, 50, 86
Caicus, river 103
Calama 74
Caracalla 76
Caria 73
Carthage 74
central nervous system (CNS) 29, 31
Chamoux, François 143
Charlier, Philippe 4
Chios 69
Chiron, centaur 39, 40, 41
chronic ailments 114
chronic diseases 84, 116, 133
Cibyra (in southern Phrygia) 53
Cicogna, PierCarla 18, 39
Cilicia 73
Classical period 1, 67, 70
Claudius, emperor 52
Clinics 51
cognition 10–15, 16, 94, 123, 139
   collective 13
   human 8, 9, 14, 15, 147, 154, 159, 160
   normative 13, 15, 115, 117
   offline 146, 147
   symbolic 107
cognitive abilities 15, 137, 154
cognitive anchors 12
cognitive approach(es) 5, 8, 9, 15, 159,
cognitive capacities 9, 10, 11
cognitive care 18, 129, 130
cognitive development 12
cognitive dissonance 152
cognitive evolution 12

cognitive governance systems 12–13
cognitive historiography 1, 8, 160
cognitive neuroscience 146
   cognitive neuroscientists 10
cognitive processing 34, 105
cognitive psychology 146
cognitive science(s) 5, 6, 8, 9, 153, 158, 159, 160
   cognitive scientists 8, 9, 10, 11, 160
cognitive theories 8, 9, 10, 15, 19, 153, 159, 160
cognitive universals 10
collective networks 12
Combs, Allan 18, 136
commonsense 157, 160
conditioning
   behavioural 30–31
   cultural 83
   negative 83, 84, 113
   Pavlovian 30
   see also deconditioning 131
conformity bias 115, 117, 156
context effects 25
Corinth 70, 72, 120
Coronis 39–40
Corpus Hippocraticum 37, 55, 57, 59, 134
counterintuitive concept(s) 7, 47, 111
counterintuitive features 61
Crete 1, 48, 70, 77
Cronus 45, 122
cult authorities 68, 115
cult centres 69, 73
cult officials 19, 117
cultural category 47, 60, 83
cultural models 13–14
cultural system(s) 10, 11, 14, 16, 54
cupping 27
   instruments 45, 86, 113
Cyclopes 40, 41
Cyllene 72
Cynno 94, 95

Cyrene 74, 97
Cyreneans 97

deafness 114
decision-making 6, 155
deconditioning 131
Deeley, Quinton 17, 91, 105
deification 41, 47, 48, 60
Delos 50, 63, 73
Delphi 63, 69, 70
depression 28, 33, 82, 84, 93
deprivation effects 145
deprivation, perceptual 144–145
deprived environment, sensory 123
despair 7, 23, 34, 35, 68, 81, 84, 89, 114
diagnosis 133, 134
Didyma (Miletos) 63
diet(s) 55, 57
dietetics 51
dieting 58
Diogenes the Cynic 97
Dionysius 53
Dionysus 45, 53
distress 23, 27, 68
divination 62–65
divine revelation(s) 65, 104, 145, 156, 158
divine signs 63–64
divine will 63, 64, 106, 127
diviners 54
doctors
   mortal 37, 42, 44, 47, 49, 140, 142, 155
   conventional 131
   Hippocratic/Hippocratics 18, 50, 55, 56, 58, 111, 119, 121, 134–136
   Homeric 45, 49
   professional/professional physicians 38, 50, 55, 59, 60, 82, 83, 91, 112, 113
   public 49, 51
Dodona (Epeirus) 63
dogs 66, 103, 106, 107
dopamine
   arousal system 104
   pathway, mesolimbic 88
   projections 107–108
   release 17, 31, 105
   secretion 104, 105
   system 100, 104, 105, 106, 108
dopaminergic activity 104
dopaminergic neurons 27
dopaminergic signals 88
dreamers 65, 136, 138, 139, 140, 142
dreaming brain 18, 123, 136, 138, 139
dreaming experiences 65, 134, 140, 142
dreaming narratives 136, 138
dreams
   Hippocratic theory of 18, 136
   divine/non-divine 65, 135–136, 146
   healing 4, 18, 19, 65–66, 75, 77, 112, 116, 123, 124, 134
   lucid 139
   oracular 65
   prognostic 135
   prophetic/non-prophetic 64–65
   sacred 146
   therapeutic 144
   waking 145
dropsy 114
drowsiness 145
drug-sellers (φαρμακοπῶλαι) 54

ecstasy 63
Egypt 71
embodied (cognition/humans/individuals/norms/organisms) 12, 14–15, 117, 159
embodied experiences 154
embodiment 11, 19, 99
embodiment theory 146
embrained (beings/cognition/humans/individuals/

organisms) 12, 14–15, 159
emotion regulation systems 13
emotional arousal 104, 156
emotional care 18, 129, 130
emotional disorders 133
emotional states 6, 14, 29
enculturation 91
encultured (beings/cognition/
    individuals) 14, 15, 159
endocrine system 30, 31
endogenous opiates 29
enhypnion (ἐνύπνιον) 65
enkoimetērion (ἐγκοιμητήριον) 77
Epeirus 63, 69
Ephesus 48, 52
epilepsy (Sacred Disease) 28, 55, 58, 114
Epione 45, 77, 127
epiphanies 127, 128
Erickson, Milton 18, 143
Erythrae (of Ionia) 98
Eryximachos 50
Euboea 73
evolution (human) 4, 10, 12, 15, 19, 32, 33 34, 154
evolutionary origins of the placebo effect 32
expectancy effect 25
expectations
    cultural 47, 54, 60, 61, 108, 111, 112, 114, 115, 157
    of healing 80, 92, 99, 109
    domain-specific 43
    intuitive 42–43, 47, 60, 61, 110–111
    manipulation of 31–32
    negative 130
    neutral 130
    outcome 94, 100
    personal 34
    positive 129, 131
    reward 87, 89, 107–108
    self-efficacy 100, 156

farmakides (φαρμακίδες) 54
fatigue 31, 33, 34, 80
fear of death 7
fear of social exclusion 23
fear of the unknown 82–84
festering sores 114
festival(s) 52, 98–99
fever 33
fountains 77
Fregellae 74

Galen 52–53, 59
games 99
Gaul 74
Geertz, Armin W. 11, 14, 16
Geertz, Clifford 13, 17, 104, 105
Gesler, Wilbert 79, 81
Gortys 72
gout 58, 92, 105, 114, 133
Greek cities 49, 71
Greek oracles 62–63
Gula of Isin 48
Guthrie, Stewart 37, 42, 62

Halieis 69
headache 28, 92, 114, 133
healers
    divine 37, 38, 49, 61, 65, 68, 70, 104, 141
    folk 55, 59, 60, 82, 91
    itinerant 55–56
    magical 57
healing
    alternatives 67, 82, 84, 89
    hypnotic 143
    interpersonal 24, 25
    miraculous 48, 79, 85, 114
    modes of 24
    natural 24, 28
    option(s) 67, 68, 86, 89, 91, 92
    religious 1, 2, 85, 159
    supernatural 60, 114, 152, 159

technological 24
wound 29
healthcare (system) 24, 33, 34, 54, 59, 60, 61, 129
health-provider(s) 24, 60, 86, 94, 155
Helieia 72
Hellenistic cities 72
Hellenistic oecumene 67
Hellenistic era/period/times 1, 16, 65, 68, 71, 98, 113, 127
Hera 48
Herakleia 69
herbs 54, 59
Hermes 103
Hermione 69, 106
Herondas 68, 94, 95, 97
Heros Iatros 49
Hesiod 37, 39, 40, 68
Hippocrates 37, 50, 51, 52, 71, 86, 129
Hippocratic Oath 46, 50
Hobson, Allan 18, 137, 138, 140
Holowchak, Andrew M. 140
Homer 37, 39, 64, 68
hope theory 92
Humphrey, Nickolas 16, 21, 28, 32–36, 101, 121, 154, 156
Hygeia 45, 46, 77, 95, 110
hypnagogic-like states 145
hypnosis 4, 144, 158
hypnotic induction states 145
hypnotic suggestibility 145
hypnotic-like experience(s) 143–144

Iamblichus 145
Iaso 46, 103
imagery 13, 45, 151, 157, 158
    auditory 138
    cognitive 145–146
    dreaming 136, 137, 138
    primed 158
    visual 44, 53
image-schemas 104

imagination 10, 130, 150, 151, 152, 158
immortality 44, 47
immune responses 28, 30, 31, 34
immune system(s) 29, 30, 31, 33, 34
impiety 40, 56
incantations 54
incarnation 66
inflammation 29
insomnia 92, 114, 133
intentionality 61–62
intervention scenario 134
interventions
    divine 7, 43, 48, 55, 57, 60, 81, 85, 106, 121
    healing 79
    medical 18, 24, 25, 30, 35, 57, 130
    miraculous 92, 113
    pharmacological 129
    placebo 32, 130
    surgical 28, 134
inventories 51
inventory lists 50
Ischys 39, 40
Isis 141
Italian peninsula 74

Johnson, Marcia 150–151

Kahn, David 18, 136
Krippner, Stanley 18, 136
Kaphyiai 69
Kapur, Shitij 17, 104–105
Keos 69
Kios 105–106
Kirrha 69
knowledge
    categorical 146–147
    embodied 145
    empirical 59, 128
    medical 49, 51
    mundane 19, 146, 147
Knidos 69

Lambaesis 74
lame(ness) 84, 106, 111, 114
Lampsakos 69
landscapes
    natural 80, 99
    therapeutic 79, 81, 96
Larisa 86
Latin provinces 74
learning 10, 13, 59
    associations 35, 48
    associative 28, 30, 31, 32, 91, 107
    cognitive 31
    cultural 83, 104, 111, 115, 155, 157
    history 93
    instrumental 87
    mechanisms 87, 91
    non-social reward-based 87
    reinforcement 88
    reward 108
    social 87, 88
Leto 40, 48
Leucippus 39, 70
Leventhal, Howard 18, 129
libations 103
Libya, Libyans 70
lice 114
LiDonnici, Lynn 109
life-narratives/autobiographical narrative 121, 150, 152
literary men 75
localization (of illness or disease) 119, 121
Lousoi in Arkadia 48
Lycia 52
Lydia 73
Lyson of Hermione 106

Macedonia 72
Machaon 39, 45
Madaurus 74
magicians 54, 55, 56, 72
Maleas 103

Marcus Aurelius 52, 95
Marcus Julius Apellas 127
meaning response 25
Media 73
medical pluralism 38, 54, 68, 82, 86, 91, 154
medical school, Hippocratic 50, 51, 71
medical training 60
medicine
    alternative 26
    Asclepian 21, 91, 108
    conventional 130
    folk 60
    herbal 41
    Hippocratic 3, 54, 113, 155
    modern 26
    mundane 113, 114, 115, 131
    professional 60, 61
    scientific 4, 27, 84
    temple 45, 53, 85, 119
memories
    autobiographical 149, 150, 152, 158
    episodic 104, 149
    false 150–152
    implicit 122, 144, 158
    residual 138, 142, 157
memory (or mnemonic) systems 30, 82, 83, 112, 142, 146
memory errors 150
memory
    semantic 118, 119
    working 107, 137
Menander 86
merchants 72, 109
Messene 39, 69, 72
meta-awareness 139
midwives (μαῖαι) 54
minimal violation 43, 44, 47
Mnemosyne 149
modality-specific systems, brain's 146–148
Morris, P. A. 93

mortality 40, 44, 84
motor systems 31
Mount Kynortion 79
Mustis 74
mute(ness) 106, 114
Mysia 73, 86
myth(s) 3, 13, 37, 39, 40, 41, 47, 53, 99
mythical narratives 37, 50
mythical saga(s) 37, 39, 40, 42, 43, 44, 60, 70
mythical story(ies) 41, 44, 47
mythical traditions 80
mythical version(s) 39, 41, 69–70
mythology, Greek 37
Mytilene 69

naloxone 29
nausea 29
neural networks 14, 15, 29, 154
neurobiology 10, 17, 117, 139
neurocognitive sciences 8
neuro-immunological systems 30
neuroscience 9, 18, 144, 146
neurotransmitters 29, 30
Nicanor 106
nocebo effects 26, 27, 31
nocebo hyperalgesia 28
nondreaming sleeping mentation 139
normative orders 14, 15
normative physics 130
Nymphs 79
Nysa 52

observation (or imitation of others) 32, 68, 87, 155
Octavian Augustus 71
offerings 50, 52, 76, 95, 96, 97, 98, 99, 103, 119, 120–121, 156
    anatomical votive/anatomical ex votos 3, 17, 47, 48, 76, 91–92, 100, 104, 119–122, 143, 150, 156
    thank- 75, 96, 119, 127

votive 48, 95, 109, 113, 115, 119, 122, 143, 156
Olympia (Peloponnese) 63
Olympian god(s) 41, 42, 45, 48
Olympus, Mount 45
omens 63, 64
oneiric reality 139
oneirocritics 140
oneiromancy 64–65
oneiros (ὄνειρος) 65
ontological category(ies) 42–43, 47, 60, 62, 157
opioids 27, 29
Orationes (Aelius Aristides' oneiric diary/ autobiographical diary) 65, 75, 114, 140–142, 145
Ovid 40, 126

paean 98
Paieon 48
pain
    chronic 81, 133
    management 29
    modulation 27
    relief 27–29
    tolerance 34
Palestine 71
Panacea 46, 103
paralyses 114
Parkinson's disease 28, 31
Paros 73
pathogen(s) 33
pattern(s) of practice 14–16, 89, 154, 159
Pausanias 37, 71, 109
pax Romana 67
perception
    actual 150–151
    aesthetic 99
    anthropomorphic 42–43, 62, 106
    embodied 141
    fleeting 138

implicit 118
metaphorical 79
sensory 27
perceptual processing 30, 146
Phaestus 71
pharmacology 113
pharmacopoeia 113
Pherai 69, 116
Philostratus 70
Phlegyas 39
Phocis 72
Phoenicia 73
Phrygia 52, 53
physes (nature) 56–57
Pindar 37, 39–40
Piraeus 50, 125, 132
placebo analgesia 27–29
placebo drama 18, 123, 130–133, 158
plague(s) 48, 64, 70, 73
plants 42, 54, 59, 113
Plato 50, 64
Plautus 86
Pliny 51
Plutarch 77
Podalirius 39, 45
Polemon of Smyrna 76
pollution 56, 57, 102–103
ponto-geniculo-occipital waves (PGO waves) 138
prayers 58, 96–97, 98, 147
pregnancies, prolonged/protracted 92, 109
pregnancy (problems) 114, 132
prehistoric period 79
Prêtre, Clarisse 4
priesthood(s) 6, 69, 98, 113
prime(s) 117–118
primed experiences 138
primed images 144, 157
priming 18, 24, 83, 117–119, 122, 156
Proclus 76, 97
prognosis(es) 60, 85, 134

prophaseis (causes) 56–57
Pseudo-Apollodorus 40
psychological implication(s) 143–144
psychoneuroimmunology (PNI)/
    psychoendoneuroimmunology (PENI) 29
psychosis 104–105
puncture 27
purgation(s) 26, 102
purifications 54, 56, 58, 77, 100–103
purifiers (καθάρται) 54, 56, 58
purity 101–103
Pythia 69, 70
Pytho 39

reality monitoring processes 151
reasoning 6, 14, 34, 146, 150, 159
    exegetical 118
    systems 10
religious ideas 7, 11, 17, 42, 43, 105
religious institution(s) 1, 3, 67, 71, 147
religious visions 19, 147, 157
Renberg, Gil 113
representations
    cultural 72
    mental 10, 104, 107, 122, 144, 158
    meta- 10
    visual 47, 148
resurrecting from death/the dead 40, 47
resurrection 60
reward system(s) 27, 88
Rhea 45
ritual settings 18, 105, 158
rituals
    collective 149
    daily 52, 74, 98
    emotionally arousing 108
    preparatory 101, 104, 144
    purification/purificatory 77, 104
    religious 10, 17, 104–105
    therapeutic 16

Robinson, Terry 17, 107
Roman Empire 52, 54, 71, 74
Roman provinces 74
Roman temples 74
root-cutters (ῥιζοτόμοι) 54
Rossi, Ernest 17, 144
Rossi, Kathryn 17, 144

sacrifices 48, 50, 52, 58, 96, 97, 98, 99, 101, 102, 103, 104, 143
sacristan(s) 95, 97, 98, 100, 119, 127, 128, 149, 150
salience 104–108
salience hypothesis, motivational 17, 104
Samos 48
Sarapis 141
Schörner, Günther 100
Scythia 73
seers 63–64
Seleukeia 71
Seleukos Nikator 71
self-awareness 139, 141
self-consciousness 35
self-deception 84
self-healing 24, 32–36, 84, 101, 130, 144, 157, 159
self-perception 149
self-reflection 137
self-regulation 129
Semele 45
sensory inputs 10, 136
sensory stimuli 31, 105, 123
serpent(s) 44, 52, 97, 107, 126
Sibylline Books 73
Sicily 74
Sicyon 72
Sidon 73
simulation mechanisms 147–148, 158
simulation process(es) 19, 145, 147
simulation(s) 147–148
slaves 73, 94, 95, 98

sleep
  nREM 18, 136, 137, 138, 139
  REM 18, 136–138
  stage of (ἐγκαθεύδω, ἐγκατακοιμάομαι) 119
sleepers 140
sleeping experiences 139
sleeping mentation, nondreaming 139
sleeping state/states of sleeping 137, 144
Smyrna 53, 141
Snyder, Charles 92
social institution(s) 11, 16
social interaction(s) 6, 13, 14, 17, 60, 68, 72, 87, 91, 115, 123, 155, 159, 160
social networks 44, 59, 115
social norms 13, 89
social psychology 146
sociality 10, 12
Socrates 97
sorcerers (γόαι) 54
Spanos, Nicholas 150
Sparta 69
spring(s) 69, 76–77, 78, 80, 81, 102, 103
statue(s) (of Asclepius) 46, 77, 86, 96, 119, 126, 141, 147
sterility 92, 114
Stertinius Xenophon 52
Stickgold, Robert 18, 138
stomach disorders 114
stomach ulcer 28
stones in the penis 114
Strabo 51, 68
study of religion 9, 10, 11
Suetonius 73
suggested information 144, 158
suggestibility/hyper-suggestibility 145
suggestion 89, 128, 143, 151, 156, 157
  auto- 143
  direct 18
  implicit 143

indirect 18, 122, 143, 156
  social 29
  therapeutic 18, 143, 144
  verbal 31
survival 34, 42, 81
Syracuse 74
Syria 71

Tarentum 74
Tartarus 40
Telesphoros 47
temenos 77, 80, 94, 95, 98, 100, 102
Thasos 69, 73
Thebes 45, 69
Themistius 75
theology 10, 56
therapeutic practices 4, 6, 8, 65, 77, 158
Thessaly 39, 68, 69
Theveste 74
Thrasymedes 77
Thuburbo Maius 74, 102
Thubursicu Numidarum 74
Tigris 71
Titane 98
Titans 45
Torone 69
traders 72
treatment
  active 134
  divine 57, 100
  medical 8, 16, 25, 36, 44
  ritual of 138
  simulation of a 26
Trikka 39, 68, 75, 86

Troezen 69
tumours 114

ulcers 92, 114
uncertainty 81–84, 89, 129
  intolerance of 82
urban settings 74, 79, 80

Varro 51
verbal communication 26, 31, 32
Versnel, Henk S. 43, 114
Veyne, Paul 7
vision (ἐνύπνιον, ὄψιν) 119
  divine dreams and 65, 146, 148
  healing dream or/and 18, 19, 65, 66, 75, 116, 123, 124, 134, 147
  religious 19, 147, 157
  therapeutic dream or 144
  waking 145
visionary states 143
visual system(s) 147–148
Vitruvius 78
votive plaques 86

wakefulness 123, 145
waking life 136
waking reality 142
waking state(s) 137–139, 144
worldview(s) 13–14, 43, 47

Xygalatas, Dimitris 108, 149

zakoros 52
Zeus 40–41, 42, 45, 47, 63, 77

www.ingramcontent.com/pod-product-compliance
Lightning Source LLC
Chambersburg PA
CBHW062025220426
43662CB00010B/1484